Praise for *Not Just Painful Periods:*

'In this essential book, Dr Liz Murray provides accurate, practical and empowering information that every woman should have access to.'
— Professor Andrew Horne, Director of Centre for Reproductive Health, University of Edinburgh; Speciality Advisor to CMO for OBGYN, Scottish Government; and President of World Endometriosis Society

'Dr Liz Murray's *Not Just a Painful Period* is a compassionate, evidence-based guide that validates the experiences of many women who may be struggling with their health that have too often been minimised. She expertly translates complex gynaecological health information into clear and practical advice. Dr Murray skilfully blends her clinical expertise with lived experience, and tackles a wide range of conditions including endometriosis and fibroids with honesty and clarity, while equipping readers with the language and confidence to seek answers, advocate for themselves and move from coping to thriving.'
— Dr Julie Hammond, MRGCP, MBBS, BSc (Hons), DRCOG, and CEO and Founder of MamAR

Not Just Painful Periods

Not Just Painful Periods

Endometriosis, Fibroids and Menstrual Health

DR LIZ MURRAY

ASTER*

First published in Great Britain in 2026 by Aster, an imprint of
Octopus Publishing Group Ltd
Carmelite House
50 Victoria Embankment
London EC4Y 0DZ
www.octopusbooks.co.uk

An Hachette UK Company
www.hachette.co.uk

The authorized representative in the EEA is Hachette Ireland,
8 Castlecourt Centre, Dublin 15, D15 XTP3, Ireland (email: info@hbgi.ie)

Copyright © Dr Liz Murray BCA(h) 2026

Distributed in the US by Hachette Book Group
1290 Avenue of the Americas, 4th and 5th Floors
New York, NY 10104

Distributed in Canada by Canadian Manda Group
664 Annette St., Toronto, Ontario, Canada M6S 2C8

All rights reserved. No part of this work may be reproduced or utilized in any form or by any means, electronic or mechanical, including photocopying, recording or by any information storage and retrieval system, without the prior written permission of the publisher.

ISBN: 978-1-80419-383-9
eISBN: 978-1-80419-384-6

A CIP catalogue record for this book is available from the British Library.

Typeset in 12/16pt Garamond Premier Pro by Six Red Marbles UK, Thetford, Norfolk.

Printed and bound in Great Britain.

13 5 7 9 10 8 6 4 2

This FSC® label means that materials used for the product have been responsibly sourced.

Disclaimer: All reasonable care has been taken in the preparation of this book but the information it contains is not intended to take the place treatment by a qualified medical practitioner. Before making any changes in your health regime, always consult a doctor. While all the therapies detailed in this book are completely safe if done correctly, you must seek professional advice if you are in any doubt about any medical condition. Any application of the ideas and information contained in this book is at the reader's sole discretion and risk.

For every woman who resigned themselves to silently suffering – thinking that their relentless, painful, heavy periods are 'just another period'. This book is dedicated to you. May you know that they are not just painful periods, and you no longer need to feel resigned.

Contents

Introduction		1
Chapter 1	Anatomy and Periods	15
Chapter 2	Know Your Flow	35
Chapter 3	Primary Dysmenorrhoea and Primary Menorrhagia	61
Chapter 4	What is Endometriosis: The Science	73
Chapter 5	Living with Endometriosis	101
Chapter 6	Getting Diagnosed with Endometriosis	121
Chapter 7	Endometriosis Management	145
Chapter 8	Endometriosis: Fertility and Pregnancy	171
Chapter 9	Fibroids: More Than Just Heavy Periods	185
Chapter 10	Adenomyosis: Not Just the Third Wheel	201
Chapter 11	Polycystic Ovary Syndrome and Primary Ovarian Insufficiency	211
Chapter 12	Menopause: More Than Just the Retirement of Our Ovaries	227
Chapter 13	Thriving Not Surviving	245
Chapter 14	Are Your Periods Healthy and Happy?	259
Glossary		267
References		273
Acknowledgements		277
Index		279

CONTENTS

About the Author   285
Further Resources   287

INTRODUCTION

Periods have, for far too long, been seen as simply a waste product, or a marker of fertility. Periods are frequently stigmatized, historically censored and as a result have become an often-misunderstood aspect of female existence. A culture of silence has long meant women have normalized what is in fact the body's way of communicating that something could be wrong.

With 90 per cent of women experiencing painful periods during their lifetime, yet the average time for a diagnosis of endometriosis ranging between 8 and 10 years, it is no wonder many women are feeling helpless. The science proves that these symptoms are more than 'just another period', yet society is a little late in acknowledging this, leading to too many women suffering silently – myself included. But not anymore.

Many of the conversations about periods – whether in social media campaigns or whispered between close friends – are confusing, oversimplified and misdirected. This can result in a cluster of chaos with life-altering implications. I wish I were being overly dramatic here, but I'm not.

The taboos around periods extend to the way menstruation is depicted in the media. Period products have only been shown in advertising campaigns in the last ten years, and even newer is the display of red instead of blue liquid. For many years, menstrual products weren't even tested using real blood – just one example of gender inequality in medical research.

Controversy around periods is an international problem, with some cultures marking women on their period as cursed, enchanted, possessed or dirty. Menstruation is even weaponized as a woman's weakness, as though the onset of a period somehow renders us irrational, emotional and incapable of articulate thought.

Periods are seen by some as the bane of a woman's life – Mother Nature's monthly punishment. To others, they're a blessing, a spiritual experience, a religious gift. Some even believe that menstruation is a curse placed on women because of Eve's sin in the Garden of Eden. For many, it's a monthly reminder of not being pregnant – either a welcome sign or a heartbreaking one, depending on the circumstances. There are even those who celebrate the arrival of their period and embrace it as a symbol of their fertility (this was never me, but I have huge admiration and awe for anyone who has a positive relationship with their periods).

Very few of us go through life without experiencing some level of discomfort due to our periods. In fact, over 90 per cent of women encounter menstrual problems at some point during their reproductive years – and these are just the women who have sought medical help.

Women are beginning to reclaim territory in both health and society, despite gender inequalities. It is a slow march, but our right to thrive and live alongside our male counterparts is finally being recognized – with still so much work to do. Yet, while we recognize that our periods should not render us lesser mortals, there remains an elephant in the room that has been allowed to grow – whispers of its presence acknowledged, but no one daring to address it:

Painful, heavy periods are not normal.

Periods are an inescapable part of life for roughly half of the population, and while we are regaining sensible ideals over the stigmas associated with them, one key aspect has yet to be formally challenged: the notion that pain and a heavy flow are part and parcel of a 'normal' period. They're not. This metaphorical elephant needs to be properly addressed, packaged and put where it rightfully belongs.

Because we have not come this far in life, claimed our right to vote and choose our careers, only to be hindered by the notion that we must struggle every month because of a misperception that our painful periods are 'normal'.

We've come this far, now let's do it properly.

INTRODUCTION

My background

Human beings have existed on Earth for around 300,000 years, yet it's only in the last (dare we say) 10 to 20 years that we, as a species, have finally begun to acknowledge the control that periods can have over our health and wellbeing. It is, quite frankly, shameful that something which governs the quality of life for around 50 per cent of the population – and inevitably impacts the other 50 per cent – has been so widely neglected in science, understanding, social acceptance and medical support. But this isn't that book. So what book is this?

Perhaps you were once, like me, a little girl with dreams of what she wanted to be when she grew up, how many children she wanted to have, a Disney-esque vision of what her life would look like. It seems incomprehensible that the dreams, plans and intentions that many of us had growing up should, in any way, be influenced by our periods. But for far too many women, despite advances in modern medicine, this is the case. I never for a moment imagined that I'd face fertility issues, have to change my career as a doctor, enter menopause in my early thirties, and have my world turned upside down because of my periods. But here we are.

For many years, I felt that life was perpetually trying to challenge me with some sadistic sense of humour; the very month I began medical school I simultaneously began life as a chronic patient. I was 18, with my entire life mapped out before me: studying to become a doctor of women's health, then get married and have children. 'Patient' was a word I used to describe those my life would revolve around within my career – not one I ever imagined would become synonymous with me.

Navigating life as a doctor alongside life as a patient with incurable, complex diseases – predominantly those affecting my gynaecological organs – for so long seemed to pose a juxtaposition of conflicting circumstances. The more I fought to advance in my career, the more my body appeared to fight back with disability after disability, and complication after complication. Everything I had planned for my future as a doctor – my lifelong ambition – was being pulled away from me. The irony was that I was destined to be a patient rather than treating patients. Or so it seemed.

Then came an epiphany. What I had for so long thought to be opposing life experiences actually proved to be a unique opportunity to have a broader impact for patients – just not in the way I had envisioned.

My life had been turned upside down by period-related health conditions: endometriosis, secondary infertility, recurrent miscarriages, surgical complications, and birth trauma. Like so many women who face gynaecological health challenges, I had experienced first-hand the impact of these things physically, mentally, on my career, and on my relationships. At times I had, like too many others, lost a sense of control over the direction of my own life – my sense of self – my ability to thrive, not just survive.

And yet, my journey was unique, having experienced it as both patient and doctor. While navigating the system as a patient, I wasn't just observing and receiving care blindly or without insight into how that system works. I was both a doctor by the bedside and a patient in the bed. So why was it that, even as a doctor facing this journey, I still encountered multiple barriers: feeling gaslit, lost, confused and far from empowered. In essence, I have reflected that so much comes down to communication, which leads to knowledge, which provides empowerment, and thus true autonomy over our health.

Autonomy over our health gives us the liberation to thrive, not just survive.

And that is my intention for this book: to provide you with the knowledge, tools and insights to bridge the ever-widening gap between patient and doctor. With patients struggling to find continuity with their GP, or even to access a GP at all, people are increasingly turning to social media and online sources for information. The danger here is that a significant amount of online information is actually misinformation, often produced by patient advocates without medical training, or AI-generated content littered with inaccuracies.

Despite what we have historically accepted through a dismissive socio-normative approach, periods are not merely markers of our fertility. Further to this, periods should not be 'the bane of a woman's life': a monthly halt to our daily plans and our ability to work or socialize. Women are finally beginning to recognize that painful, heavy periods are not normal, and here I present the medically reliable information so desperately needed by so many.

Periods can be everything for women, but they should dictate nothing.

Their arrival marks the onset of our fertile phase of life. The transition from childhood into puberty can be turbulent as we are introduced to our new sense of self, and our lives become very much influenced and regulated by our sex hormones. As we progress through our prime years we make plans – but our ovaries, hormones and uterus don't always receive the message and make plans of their own. Then the transition into 'fertility retirement' as we enter menopause brings us to a sort of puberty-in-reverse.

The underlying cells, hormones and organs behind our monthly periods are functioning to a steady beat of instructions laid down over millions of years of evolution, dictating that we should be (with an often-unwanted reminder) reproductive primal beings. While at our cellular core we cannot deny this, it does not for one moment mean that any part of these processes has the right to dominate, dictate or claim ownership of our lives. The right to thrive remains ours and ours alone. We have not collectively fought for our right to vote and begun liberating ourselves from a patriarchal society, only to stop short of liberating ourselves from our periods.

Your identity

A period is something you have, not something by which you should be governed. Your identity should not be a labelled an 'endo warrior' or 'fibroid warrior', nor should you feel you have lost your sense of self as you enter menopause. In short, your identity should not become a diagnosis.

I, like many menstruating women, spent far too many years believing that my painful and heavy periods were normal. That my difficulty adapting and coping with the severity of the pain, the flooding through three nighttime pads during the day, and the time off work were simply signs of my own inability to cope. I had never been taught to recognize my periods as a marker of my gynaecological health rather than just a marker of my fertility. Just as we, as women, are more than walking incubators with a reserve of eggs-in-waiting, our gynaecological organs and processes are a core part of us as healthy, living, functioning beings with desires, emotions and drives. This should not be new information, but if this lands as a lightbulb moment or validating epiphany you never knew you needed, you're welcome. It wasn't until I was in my late thirties that I found out just how much my periods were a marker of my overall health. This late discovery left me facing the uncertainty of gynaecological disease made worse by late diagnosis, poor compliance with proposed treatments and IVF that was destined to fail. Which raises the question – why am I writing this book?

Why I wrote this book

It can take something catastrophic to happen before failings reveal themselves in full, which then allow a system to rebuild stronger. The process of reflection and the beauty of hindsight is what brought me to write this book.

Having experienced a whole spectrum of women's health conditions while working as a medical doctor for over ten years, I eventually realized that I had fallen through far too many gaps in the system. After being left with complications of mismanaged endometriosis – bowel and bladder damage, £12,000 ($16,000 USD) lost to IVF that was never appropriate, six miscarriages and an early hysterectomy – I reached a point where I was forced to stop and reflect. If this happened to me as a doctor, a woman with insider knowledge who theoretically knew the warning signs of period-related disease, how to navigate the system and advocate for myself, what chance did other women have?

As I began to rebuild life – physically, professionally and emotionally – I took a step back to take stock. In order to figure out where it had gone wrong, I needed to understand why, despite my medical training, I was so misguided that I wasn't able to diagnose myself. Had I missed the lesson on listening to your period as a warning sign of gynaecological health? After I was finally diagnosed with endometriosis, hadn't I listened to the counselling on the true nature, impact and complexity of this disease? Why didn't I have the knowledge that might have empowered me to make the right choices for myself? In fact, I didn't miss those things: they were never there.

Even now, as I write this book, sex education in schools places more weight on how to use a condom than preserving gynaecological health and fertility. There is a plethora of period health advocacy online, but it is largely presented by patient-led advocates without medical qualifications. A diagnosis does not a qualification make, and with the rise of AI and Dr Google, we now face a wealth of misinformation – mostly well-intentioned but contributing to what I fear is becoming a period problem pandemic.

Women deserve knowledge: reliable medical knowledge.

We, as a cohort of menstruating women, are finally beginning to recognize that painful and heavy periods are not normal. Furthermore, we are beginning to recognize that using the word 'normal' in reference to our periods is a slippery slope where warning signs of disease are normalized, often because, for some of us, those symptoms have been present since our very first period.

It's no wonder that, while we've finally been liberated with the freedom to talk about our periods, this newfound ability to speak has come with no guidance to properly identify what it is we actually want to say. Everyone is in a room staring at this elephant, casting side glances at one another, saying, 'Okay, this shouldn't be here . . . but what do we do?'

This is why I am writing this book: to address the elephant in the room, and to dare to use my experience as both a medical doctor and a patient with lived experience of multiple women's health issues as authority to finally tackle it.

What this book will cover

This book's message could be captured in a single statement: heavy and painful periods are not normal. My aim is to first help you to understand what is happening in your own body, why so many of us experience heavy or painful periods, and the options available to you going forwards.

I want to shift away from using the phrase 'normal period' toward the better – and potentially lifesaving – term: 'healthy period'. Think about it for a moment. Doctors use urine to assess health status (volume, colour, and the presence of glucose, proteins or white cells to detect infection). We examine stool samples for blood, consistency and bacteria. We even collect mucus from our chests to better understand a patient's condition. Yet our periods are still considered mere sanitary waste – a simple monthly loss with no bearing on our health status. This is wrong.

Finally, the medical industry worldwide is beginning to recognize that our periods are markers of overall health. Who knows, maybe one day they'll even use menstrual samples to help identify underlying diseases (you heard it here first!).

The truth is that periods are a marker of our health, particularly our gynaecological health. They are not waste products to go unnoticed, tolerated or dismissed. Women have felt this intuitively for a long time, and now, finally, it is being acknowledged.

What you need now is to understand how to listen to your periods – to interpret what they're telling you about your underlying health – for the ultimate purpose of regaining control over your life. Our right as women is to thrive, not just survive. Our right is to live with periods, not be dictated by them.

Periods matter – but let's make sure this is for the right reasons.

I want you to know your flow. To do this, I'll begin by taking you back to the basics: understanding not just what periods are, but why they happen. When we grasp the processes behind menstruation, particularly the powerful influence of our hormones, we become better equipped to use that knowledge – especially when things go wrong.

If we don't have a solid understanding of what a healthy period should be – its purpose and what 'normal' looks like – we can't recognize when our periods begin to whisper, or even scream, that something is wrong. This is essential, because for some of us our periods have been screaming the warning signs of disease since puberty. Yet misleading menstrual product messaging has encouraged us to believe these warning signs are simply part of a 'normal period'.

From there, we'll explore the ways periods deviate from 'healthy', how these changes can indicate underlying disease and when they signal problems that shouldn't be impacting our lives. Along the way, we'll address some myths around periods. One major misconception is that if painful and heavy periods are not normal, then pain and heavy bleeding must always mean disease (incorrect). Many women will discover that the cause of their painful or heavy periods is 'primary'. Primary dysmenorrhoea and primary menorrhagia are not disease processes in the obvious sense; nothing is anatomically wrong. Primary causes of pain or heavy bleeding are a result of the menstrual cycle being dysfunctional rather than due to a secondary disease. This is something I explain in detail through the book and is a vital piece of the puzzle, one that I believe could help empower women who do not receive an anticipated diagnosis, such as endometriosis.

I'll then outline the key underlying period-related disorders, debunk the myths and present clear guidance on recognizing your symptoms, getting diagnosed and managing these conditions. Many of you reading this will already know that anything related to periods and hospital referrals is a slow process, but here's the newsflash: many of these conditions can be managed by your GP. And while I recognize that even accessing a GP appointment can feel like another barrier, equipping yourself with as much information and as many tools as possible will help you move faster, stronger and more confidently through the system, and even dodge a few hurdles along the way. Because knowledge is power, power gives us autonomy and autonomy is the key to shifting from surviving to thriving.

A large part of this book will focus on endometriosis. As a patient, I loathe the condition for the relentless, brutal and sneaky (insert curse word here) thing that it is. As a doctor, I am part intrigued by its immense complexity, part in awe of how such a disease functions.

Endometriosis is, of all gynaecological diseases, probably the most misunderstood and misrepresented in the online space. This is largely due to a lack of reliable medical voices representing the condition adequately, and too much misinformation shared by misguided patient advocates who lack medical training. Endometriosis is one of the most complex gynaecological diseases, and for too long has lacked someone who understands its nuances to discuss it with clarity (until now). This is why there are more pages devoted to endometriosis than to other conditions. Having fallen victim to its advanced form myself, I know how vital it is that this disease is explained clearly and accurately so that women can regain control of their bodies and their lives.

Of course, I'll also cover the other equally important conditions – fibroids, adenomyosis and PCOS – along with fertility, menopause and mood. A common companion throughout will be the subject of hormones. Hormones are not just silent messengers within our bodies; as you'll come to see, they influence the very essence of who we are. We may think we have free will, but that will is often directed by what our hormones want our bodies to do. When we introduce additional hormones through treatments or contraceptive pills, the impact extends far beyond the pelvis. Understanding this helps us make informed decisions about our options, treatments and ultimately our lives.

Across society, there remains a powerful, collective need among women to have the severity of their menstrual experiences acknowledged. The terms 'heavy and painful' and 'normal' have become emotionally charged, even triggering. There is still a palpable sense of injustice. After years of societal gaslighting – where women have been expected to tolerate disabling pain or excessive bleeding – the need for recognition, validation and to simply be listened to is deeply real.

For many, learning about the 'big three' conditions – fibroids, adenomyosis and endometriosis – feels like long-overdue vindication, as though finally there is a name for what they've silently endured for years. But what's often missing in this conversation is the understanding that a period disorder is significant and valid, regardless of whether it stems from one of these three specific diagnoses.

Gynaecological cancers

This book mostly focusses on the non-malignant gynaecological diseases. Gynaecological cancers are a book within themselves, and the purpose of these chapters is to educate and empower you to manage period-related conditions. There are times when I have highlighted where a symptom could indicate an underlying malignancy (for example, the return of bleeding after menopause, see page 230), and anyone experiencing a sudden change in bleeding pattern at any life stage, whether accompanied by other red flag symptoms or not, should seek medical attention.

Who this book is for

This is the book I wish I had been given when I entered puberty. Had I been equipped with even some of the insights I share in the first few chapters, the entire trajectory of my life would have been different. Had I been given this book in my early twenties, I could have used so much of the guidance and the toolkits to navigate my endometriosis journey very differently. Had I been presented with this book when I had my hysterectomy for advanced endometriosis, I would have approached early menopause with far more confidence and positivity and felt empowered to make informed decisions for myself.

I've tried to capture within one book all the knowledge and tools menstruating women need to regain control over their lives. Within these pages you'll discover what a healthy period is (or should be), learn how to listen to your body and get to know your flow, so you can recognize when something isn't right.

From that foundation, this book provides medically accurate, reliable information from someone who knows and appreciates the realities of these symptoms, procedures and treatments, along with toolkits and guidance to help you navigate not only the healthcare system, but also the wider impact on your life. More importantly, it's here to help you mitigate that impact and regain, restore and reclaim ownership of your life.

Some of these insights may be entirely new. Some of you reading this may already have a sense that something is 'off' but aren't sure where to go for information or what to do next. Wherever you are on your journey, you're likely beginning to realize that periods are not a mere passenger in your life – they are a core part of your health and wellbeing. As such, I want this book to be your starting point for empowerment.

'Women'

I recognize and validate that what we commonly refer to as a 'woman' is not defined by genetics, the presence of specific gynaecological organs or the experience of menstruation. There are women who identify as women but were born without these organs. There are women with these organs who do not menstruate. There are women who menstruate but cannot conceive. And there are people who have these organs but do not identify as women.

When I use the word 'woman' in this book, it is not to exclude anyone – quite the opposite. My intention is to provide knowledge, tools and empowerment to anyone who menstruates. I use 'woman' as a biological descriptor, not a boundary.

My intention

I have exercised due diligence and commitment to ensure that the information on these pages is informed by the latest medical research, guidelines and knowledge available to me at the time of writing. As an advocate for reliable patient education and the regulation of online health information, I take this responsibility seriously. The references and guidance I use align with the clinical standards and evidence-based practices I was trained in at medical school.

INTRODUCTION

> This book is not prescriptive; it is an informed guideline, a companion filled with information, insight and practical tools. The examples and recommendations of how things should happen in hospitals or GP practices are based on national guidance and clinical best practice.

Before we begin...

As you move through these pages, remember why you picked up this book in the first place: like many women everywhere, you recognize the elephant in the room.

You should not be faced each month with just another painful period. Periods should be healthy and not disrupt your quality of life. You have the right to be liberated from painful, heavy periods and to reclaim your ability to thrive as an independent woman.

We have fought far greater battles than this and we have won. Now it's time to reclaim the right to live as women free from the control of our periods, or at the very least, to recognize our periods for what they are: markers of our health, not the measure of our worth.

CHAPTER 1:
ANATOMY AND PERIODS

UNDERSTANDING YOUR PERIODS

Periods are more than a monthly reminder of our biological sex. They are a marker of our health and we need to learn how to listen to them.

- Period
- Time of the month
- Monthly visit from Mother Nature
- Flow is in town
- The decorators are in
- Aunt Flo
- Monthlies
- The Curse
- On the Blob

However you refer to yours, there is no escaping the palpable presence (or absence) in a woman's life of her period. Periods are far more than the marker of our fertility, an indication of our biological sex or a reminder of our primal purpose to reproduce. Periods, or more accurately the underlying physiological and physical processes which regulate and dictate them, inform the essence of who we are, how we behave and our body's wellbeing. If something in this process is disrupted, every aspect of our life can be profoundly impacted. In order to begin exploring the ways in which periods *can go wrong* and present problems for us, we need to understand what they are, why we have them and the role of oestrogen and progesterone.

What are periods?

The scientific answer is that periods are a biological marker of reproductive health. Aside from the archaic beliefs that periods are some divine curse – a punishment handed down to Eve's descendants for eating the forbidden apple – they are, in essence, a by-product of the intricate hormonal processes that make us reproductive human beings. As a mammalian species we have evolved with hard-wired DNA coding to do two things: survive and reproduce. This survival-reproduction model is split across the two biological sexes, each with vastly different roles in the reproductive process (one might even say it is grossly unequal in its division).

The fact that we have evolved to a point where reproduction is often a choice, a privilege or even a luxury is absolutely worth celebrating. Our modern lives no longer demand that we hunt, gather or physically fend off predators to survive. In much of the Western world we're privileged to (in many senses) live without the daily threats that distinguish us from humans that existed 100,000 years ago. But at our cellular core, our bodies have not forgotten their evolutionary programming. That primal instinct for survival and reproduction is still very much in place. This matters, because forgetting that much of our behaviour, emotions, responses, desires and even ambitions are influenced by this primal undercurrent is to overlook something essential about what it means to be human.

So how does this relate to periods? To survive and reproduce, women's bodies have evolved an intricate, complex system of hormones and biological drivers. The true extent to which these processes influence our bodies – physically, mentally and the essence of who we are and how we behave – is greater than many of us may realize.

Women's bodies are designed to become fertile in adolescence, affording us around 20 to 30 years of reproductive potential before entering menopause, putting us into reproductive retirement. Periods are just a small cog in the machinery of fertility, but one that has a potentially monumental impact on our quality of life.

Why do we have periods?

Periods are a by-product of being reproductive beings, that is beings that are biologically hard-wired to sustain the human species. Understanding the 'why' is crucial because the hormones that govern our periods influence far more than just when we bleed. If we think about how period-related disorders like endometriosis are only recently being recognized, we've barely scratched the surface. The tidal wave of understanding around hormones as influencers of our mental and physical wellbeing hasn't yet fully landed. The role hormones play in driving the menstrual cycle is profoundly influential. Knowing that these processes are hard-wired and rooted in primal biological imperatives is not a trivial detail (see page 29 for more on this).

Understanding these elements opens the floodgates to a powerful toolkit – one that allows us to see how every decision we make in response to our periods, particularly around hormonal contraception or treatments for menstrual disorders, directly shapes who we are and how we feel. Understanding this can be liberating and restore our quality of life.

It may sound dramatic, but that's because it is. These groundbreaking scientific insights have not always been properly communicated to many people. It's information I was robbed of for years, both as a doctor and as a patient, with devastating consequences to my fertility, organ preservation and quality of life. As a woman I feel it a moral duty to empower others, and as a mother of a daughter I would not want her going through life experiencing the same blind-folded puppetry I did. As a medical professional I truly believe that patients have a right to truly informed consent, and this means being presented with all the facts and information.

As these concepts and information leap off the page, my hope is that everything starts to make sense to you and you realize that you *do* have choices. You *can* have control over your own period health. And suddenly, the suffering and struggles you once thought were inevitable . . . start to look very different.

FEMALE ANATOMY

For us to understand what a healthy period looks and feels like, it is important to have an awareness of the key players in this process. Let's think of the reproductive system as an orchestra where the instruments (the organs) are affected by multiple conductors (the hormones) and each have roles to ensure the symphony plays without a hitch. This orchestra is more complex than most, as there are multiple conductors (hormones) that step forward and back in response to one another depending on what stage of the symphony is active. If a fault in the orchestra arises, we need to understand how each element works in order to understand what the problem is. Likewise, one wrong note doesn't mean the entire symphony is broken, but it also shouldn't be ignored.

It's also important to know that some of the body's processes don't just stay within the theatre of the reproductive system; they can have a wider impact on the body as a whole.

> As with any mechanistic process, the more moving parts, the more the potential for things to go wrong. Our hormones should not be dismissed as simply 'silent messengers' in the menstrual cycle. Their powers extend far beyond the uterus and ovaries, and have major implications for mood-related disorders and hormone-based treatments (see pages 152–62 for more on this).

In many cultures, a certain discomfort exists around using the correct terminology for women's organs. This stems in part from the oversexualization of the female body, which has led to embarrassment, miscommunication and knowledge gaps. If we don't know the proper names for our own body parts, how can we possibly describe symptoms clearly to a healthcare professional? In the words of Harry Potter: 'Fear of a name increases fear of the thing itself.'

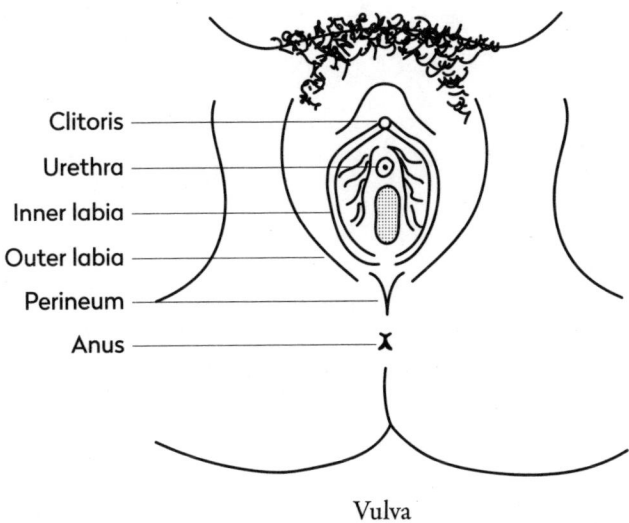

Vulva

By avoiding accurate terms like 'vagina' or 'vulva', we do ourselves a great disservice. If we truly want to be empowered when it comes to our health, we must first learn to speak the same anatomical language as our doctors. So, if by the end of this chapter you realize you didn't know the difference between your vagina and your vulva, please don't worry. You're not alone.

At the centre of our gynaecological system is the **uterus**, also referred to by some as the womb. The uterus is a muscular, balloon-shaped organ that prepares to receive and nurture a pregnancy. It is where the menstrual lining builds up and sheds from during a period, and where contractions occur during labour. Because the uterus is actively working at a cellular level every day in response to multiple processes, it is inevitable that sometimes things go wrong just the same as any other organ. The uterus doesn't just sit quietly waiting until it is given its 'shining moment' with a pregnancy. It is actively changing and responding to our hormones every single day. Like any other organ, the uterus is not immune to problems arising.

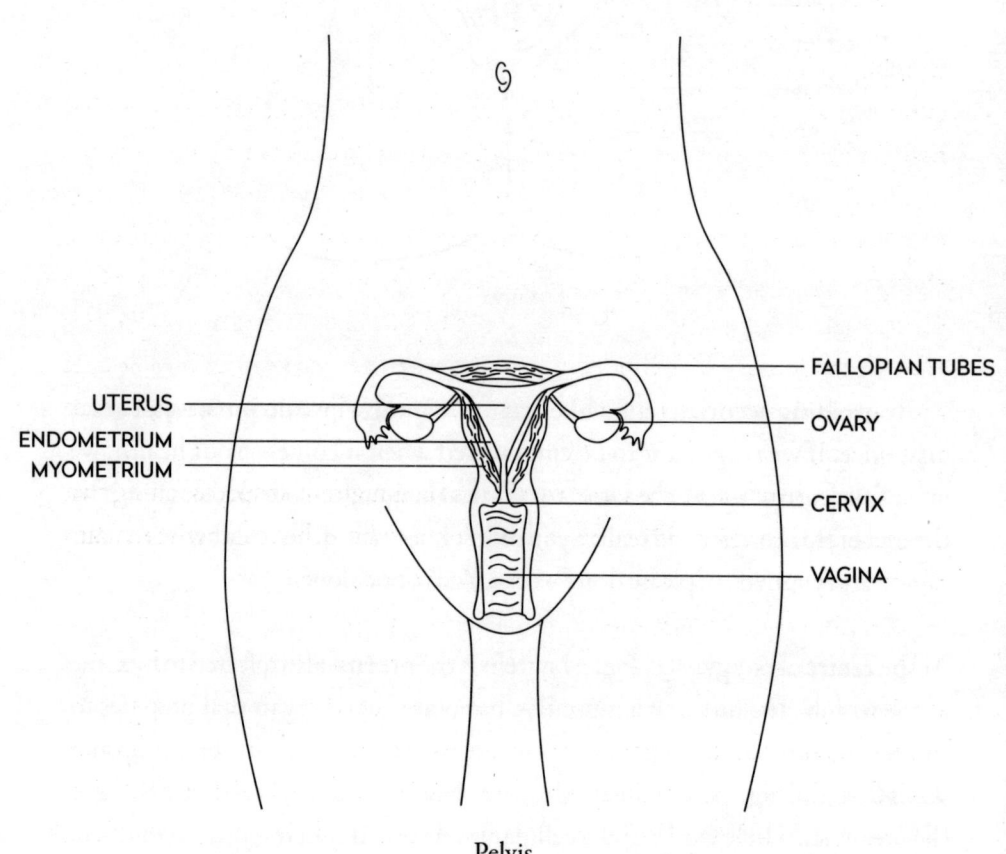

Pelvis

> Fun fact: the ovaries are not actually fixed to the fallopian tubes. They 'float' nearby, attached to the uterus by a ligament. The finger-like ends of the fallopian tubes hover around the ovaries, ready to guide the released egg into the tube.

Branching out from the uterus are the **fallopian tubes** – slender tubes that extend toward the ovaries, ending in delicate, finger-like projections that help guide the egg into the tube. Nestled nearby the ends of the tubes are the **ovaries**, which house a woman's eggs. Women are born with all the eggs they'll ever have, their quantity and genetic make-up pre-determined before their own birth. When a pregnant woman carries a girl, she is also carrying all the eggs her baby will ever have. In essence, she's carrying part of her future grandchild – an extraordinary fact I still find fascinating! Female eggs are finite and age with us, which differs from men, who continuously produce new sperm.

At the base of the uterus is the **cervix**, a soft, doughnut-shaped opening that connects to the vagina. The cervix dilates during labour, but otherwise remains a narrow opening that allows menstrual blood out and sperm in.

The **vagina** and the **vulva** are the two most confused parts. The vagina is the internal canal – the part you cannot see – where a tampon is inserted. The vulva, on the other hand, is made up of everything you *can* see externally: the labia, the clitoris and the vaginal opening. Many people confuse these terms, using them interchangeably without realizing they describe different parts of the anatomy.

Understanding the difference is essential because each of these six main structures is vulnerable to specific diseases and cancers. The six main gynaecological cancers are:

- Fallopian tubes
- Ovaries
- Uterus

- Cervix
- Vagina
- Vulva

All these organs sit within the pelvis and work together to make reproduction possible. Each month, they respond to hormonal signals that prepare the body for pregnancy. If pregnancy does not occur, the cycle resets and the uterus sheds its lining – a process we know as a period. This monthly rhythm is driven by hormones: *our periods are governed by hormones acting on specific reproductive structures*. While many hormones are involved, the two primary players are oestrogen and progesterone, the key drivers of this cyclical process.

THE STAGES OF WOMANHOOD

The 'stages' in a woman's life are often oversimplified as:

1. **Pre-puberty**: Childhood, before our gynaecological organs are stimulated by hormones and begin to dominate much of our lives.
2. **The fertile years:** From the first period until menopause.
3. **Menopause**: The end of menstruation.

In reality, a woman's life is marked by several distinct stages and milestones, all influenced by the reproductive system.

1. **Childhood**: The early years before the sex hormones begin to truly 'set in'.
2. **Puberty**: This stage begins when breast buds start to form, signalling the onset of puberty. There are physical changes with the female body such as a curvier shape, pubic hair starting to grow and the distinctive body odour smell. Hormonal changes start 2–3 years before the first period, and girls can begin experiencing monthly mood fluctuations from as early as eight years old. Without awareness of what's happening, families may feel confused or frustrated by a young girl who seems to be 'crying

for no reason'. This is a crucial window for education: girls should be taught what's coming, so they can understand and feel empowered by the changes to their bodies.
3. **Menarche**: This is the medical term for a girl's first period. It usually occurs around age 11 or 12, though it can happen earlier (before the age of eight should warrant medical investigation) and usually by the age of 16 (if not, see your doctor). In the years following menarche, the menstrual cycle often takes time to 'regulate' and find its own rhythm. This doesn't necessarily mean early warning signs such as heavy or severely painful periods should be ignored. Conditions like endometriosis can begin to present themselves during this time.

Puberty

It is scientifically recognized that the onset of puberty is happening at an earlier age, though the underlying cause is unknown. It is now not uncommon for girls to start puberty at the age of eight. By starting puberty I mean the onset of body changes (pubic hair growth, breasts developing) in response to hormonal shifts preparing us to become reproductively viable adults. Twenty years ago, this would prompt medical investigations, but it is now considered normal.

---

4. **Fertile Years**: The many decades that span from menarche to menopause are typically characterized by regular cycles, hormonal fluctuations, mood swings and the ever-present societal pressure of the 'ticking clock'. This phase can last several decades and is often the most discussed, yet still poorly understood, part of a woman's reproductive life.
5. **Perimenopause**: Menopause doesn't just begin overnight. Perimenopause is the transition phase leading up to menopause and can begin as early as age 35. Many women are unaware that it can start without

any changes to their periods. Symptoms such as hot flushes, mood shifts, memory lapses and fatigue can quietly creep in. Without context, women may start to question their mental health, their relationships, even their careers – never realizing that they are amid a natural hormonal transition. Just as puberty is the body's shift into fertility, perimenopause is the body's shift out of it.

6. **Menopause**: Defined as the point at which a woman hasn't had a period for 12 consecutive months, menopause marks the official end of the reproductive years. It's a milestone that should be acknowledged and supported with care, not just brushed off as a footnote in a woman's life.

7. **Post-menopause:** This is the stage that follows menopause and lasts for the rest of a woman's life. Depending on the age at which menopause occurred, the severity of symptoms and whether hormonal support is needed, this phase can bring profound physical, emotional and psychological changes. For many women, it is as significant a transition as puberty.

Without a clear understanding of these stages – and particularly the hormonal and physical changes they bring – women are left ill-equipped to interpret what's happening in their own bodies. I've met countless women who believed they were 'losing their minds', questioning their relationships, careers, even their sanity, only to discover they had unknowingly entered perimenopause in their thirties. No one had told them this was even possible. But when people understand why things are happening – when they have context and language – they can begin to make sense of the changes, regain control and navigate their health with confidence rather than fear or confusion.

POWERHOUSE HORMONES

The operation of monthly menstruation is a complex mechanism between organs and hormones. Hormones are the 'directors' of the process, influencing the priming and releasing and preparing of our eggs for fertilization. Each month the system must prepare for the possibility of a pregnancy, being ready to quickly switch into pregnancy mode. If a pregnancy doesn't occur, the body hits the reset button and the process starts all over again.

First, **GnRH** (gonadotropin-releasing hormone) is produced by the brain to instruct the pituitary gland to release LH (luteinizing hormone) and FSH (follicle-stimulating hormone). Essentially the GnRH is the first part of the relay race and kick-starts the second messengers (the LH and FSH).

LH and **FSH** have very active roles in travelling down to the ovaries to signal oestrogen and progesterone to 'do their part'. They are the lesser-acknowledged key players without which oestrogen and progesterone could not function.

Oestrogen and progesterone: the dynamic duo

The two hormones with significant influence driving this entire process – oestrogen and progesterone – play distinct but interconnected roles. Each is equally vital in orchestrating the complex cycle of monthly menstruation and, while they function independently, if one goes rogue, the other can't function properly. While they work in tandem, their presence within the body is felt very differently.

Oestrogen is the hormone most people associate with the female body. While men do have some oestrogen (just as women have some testosterone), oestrogen is considered the predominant 'female' hormone. We can think of oestrogen as the Chief Executive Officer (CEO) and progesterone as the Chief Operating Officer (COO) of the female reproductive system.

Oestrogen is responsible for initiating the menstrual cycle. It encourages the ovaries to prepare for ovulation, stimulates the endometrium to begin thickening and sends signals throughout the body to prepare itself. As oestrogen levels rise in the first half of the cycle, the brain also registers these changes, often influencing mood, memory and motivation. Oestrogen acts as the project manager or director of operations for the reproductive system.

Progesterone, on the other hand, takes over after ovulation. Its role is to maintain the thickened endometrium and prepare the body for a potential pregnancy. If an embryo implants successfully, progesterone remains high and becomes the dominant hormone throughout pregnancy. It suppresses further ovulation by keeping oestrogen levels in check. If no pregnancy occurs, progesterone levels drop, the endometrial lining is shed and the cycle begins again – handing the reins back to oestrogen.

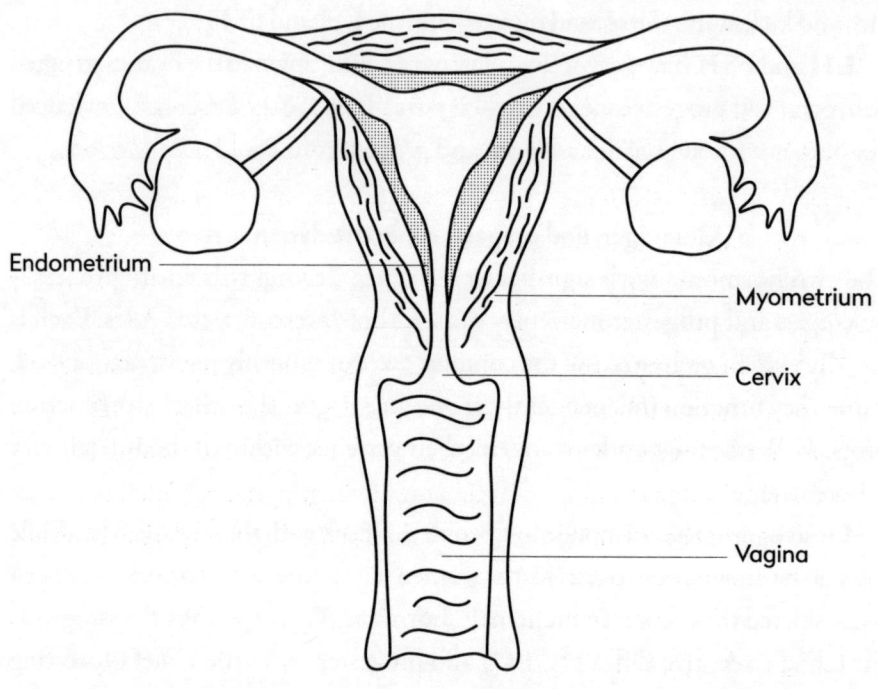

Uterus with endometrium

THE ENDOMETRIUM

The uterus has two main layers: a muscular layer called the myometrium and an inner layer known as the endometrium. The myometrium is responsible for contractions – contracting to expel a period and, if a pregnancy occurs, contracting to push a baby out through the cervix and vagina during labour. The endometrium is the layer that undergoes changes throughout the monthly cycle and is directly involved in menstruation.

The endometrium has two sub-layers:

- A **basal (base) layer**, which remains constant and never sheds.
- A **functional layer**, which thickens in response to hormonal signals and is shed during menstruation if pregnancy does not occur.

As the cycle progresses and ovulation approaches, the endometrium thickens, creating ideal conditions for an embryo to implant. If fertilization and implantation occur, the body switches into 'pregnancy mode'. If not, hormone levels drop sharply, triggering the shedding of the endometrial lining – this is what becomes the menstrual period. This build-up of the uterine lining is a crucial part of the cycle and central to understanding period disorders.

A period is made up of blood, endometrial tissue and vaginal secretions. This is why clots can sometimes be seen; if the tissue takes time to exit the body, it may begin to clot before leaving through the vagina. The colour and consistency of menstrual flow often change depending on the stage of the period; it may start pink and watery, become bright red during the heaviest flow and darken to brown as the blood ages toward the end.

OVULATION

During each monthly cycle, the ovaries must prepare a small group of eggs for possible ovulation. These aren't fully developed eggs; they're called oocytes, immature eggs that need to ripen to allow for fertilization to occur. Women are born with far more oocytes than they will ever use in their lifetime. These eggs remain in a dormant, 'hibernating' state within the ovaries until hormonal signals trigger them to awaken.

Each month, various hormones encourage a handful of oocytes to begin maturing. Of these, usually only one becomes the 'chosen one' and is released during ovulation, travelling down the fallopian tube in hopes of being fertilized by sperm and forming an embryo. While multiple eggs may begin to mature, only

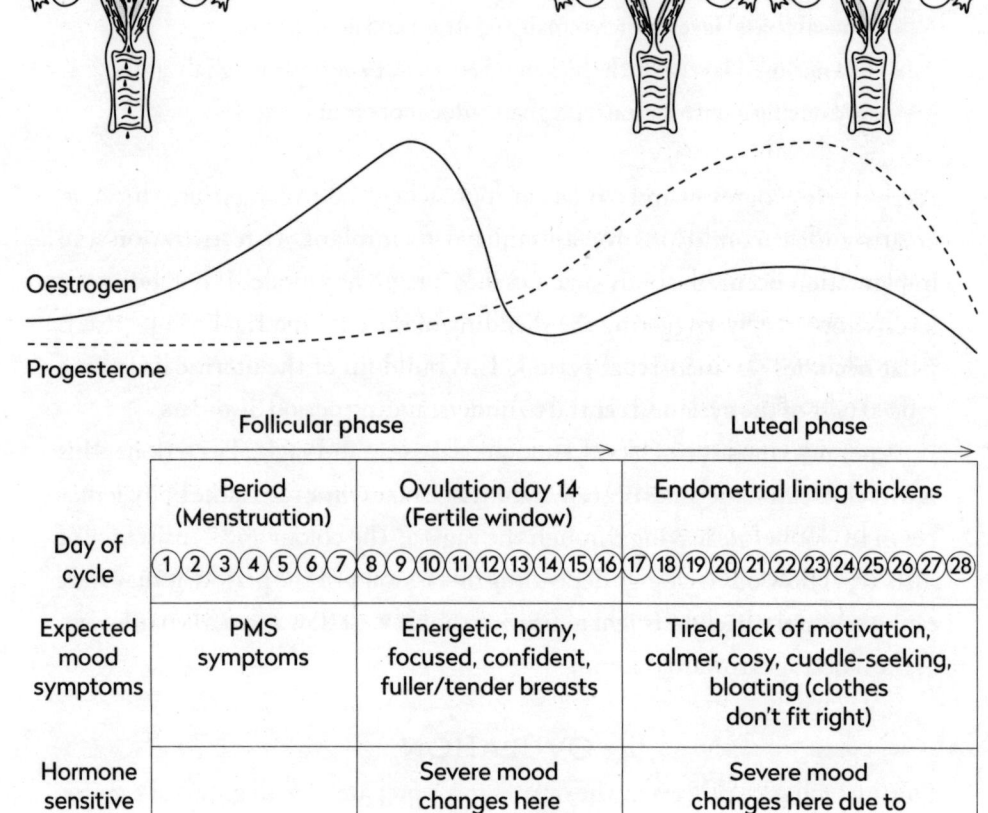

The 28-day menstrual cycle

one typically makes it to ovulation (occasionally more than one egg is released, which can result in twins). The body tightly regulates this process, aiming to select and fully commit to just one egg each cycle.

The egg's journey doesn't end at ovulation. Once released, it is caught by the fallopian tube and slowly travels toward the uterus. If it meets sperm along the way, the egg becomes fertilized and continues onward to implant in the uterus, establishing a pregnancy.

The entire menstrual cycle takes place over 28 days (on average). It is entirely normal for some women's cycle to vary by a few days, and most women become familiar with what their individual cycle looks like. There are many charts available that show the rise and fall of different hormones over those 28 days, and I admit that even as a medical student it took me a while to remember them, particularly when they include all the hormones such as LH and FSH. What I have produced here is the chart I wish I'd had from my very first period. To make things easier I have removed the LH and FSH curves and simplified it to show when and what oestrogen and progesterone are doing. These are important to show because, for some women, the sudden drop of oestrogen can trigger immense anxiety for a day or two as the body recalibrates. For other women, it is the steady and sustained high level of progesterone that causes depression.

By having an awareness of what your hormones are doing during those 28 days, it can help to match symptoms such as pain or changes in mood with what is happening underneath. Knowing whether you personally struggle with mood symptoms around days 10–14 can help identify a sensitivity to oestrogen, while feeling depressed just before your period may suggest a sensitivity to progesterone. This information can really help you make informed choices about hormonal contraceptives and which ones you may be better suited to.

Why do humans have periods?

Every living creature needs a process of reproduction for survival, but very few species shed the unused endometrium in the form of a period – in most mammals, this is re-absorbed. The science behind why humans have evolved to do this is still in debate, with favour leaning on reasons pertaining to us as a species being more selective over our pregnancies than other mammals.

Unlike most other mammals, humans have evolved to reproduce less and invest more of our energy (for survival and living) on fewer offspring. A woman's body has to commit nine months of her life to carrying and growing a new human and so it must be certain that the embryo is strong and worth investing in (of course, this happens at cellular level without any conscious awareness from the mother).

Far more eggs are fertilized than we may realize. Nearly half of all fertilised eggs (embryos) don't make it and are rejected by the uterus. Around 30–40 per cent of these are rejected before implantation, or before a woman even realizes she is pregnant. This evolutionary process is designed to ensure that the 'chosen' embryo will be strong enough to justify the impact on, and investment by, the mother.

Some of these fertilized eggs are further 'screened' at implantation. The thickened endometrium is a nesting place for the fertilized embryo, but it is quite inhospitable and only accepts the strong and committed embryos. Even if implantation does occur, if the embryo doesn't release enough hCG (human chorionic gonadotropin – the pregnancy hormone) to signal to the rest of the organs that pregnancy has occurred, the lining will shed regardless, possibly before a woman realizes she is pregnant (this process is sometimes referred to as a chemical pregnancy). Therefore, the shedding of a period may be a way of selectively filtering out potentially unviable embryos.

To women reading this who are struggling with fertility, realizing that our bodies are hard-wired to be selective of embryos may land with some discomfort. As someone who has experienced six miscarriages and encountered secondary infertility, I understand how difficult it is to discover that 50 per cent of potential pregnancies are rejected. And when we factor in that of the 50 per cent that *do* become 'successful' pregnancies another 25 per cent are lost as a miscarriage, we begin to realize just how difficult it can be to become pregnant.

> But remember that our fertility is part of a long-built evolutionary process spanning over 300,000 years with deep-rooted mechanisms influenced by our survival instincts as a species. Some of these processes are far beyond our control.

HORMONAL IMPACT

Scientists are just beginning to recognize the widespread outreach of oestrogen and progesterone, and they hold a lot more power than we previously gave them credit for.

Physical attraction

Oestrogen, the bossy CEO in charge of encouraging egg production and fertilization, has a role that extends beyond the uterus. To signal to the woman (and potential mating partner) that she is 'fertile', oestrogen receptors around the body detect the rising oestrogen and respond accordingly, for example causing our breasts to swell and become tender. Oestrogen is responsible for our 'womanly curves', biologically designed to signal fertility to a mating partner. It also influences our libido and energy levels. Recent studies have shown that women are attracted to different male physiques depending on where they are in their monthly cycle, i.e. how high or low their oestrogen is. When the body is preparing for optimum fertilization, women are more likely to be more drawn to the strong, testosterone-associated male who biologically signals a 'safe bet' for fertility (this is a scientific phenomenon, not a stereotype here – don't shoot the messenger!). Whereas during the 'nesting' phase of the cycle when a woman's progesterone levels are high and the uterus is hopefully embedding a pregnancy, a woman is more likely to be drawn to a man who appears safe, protective and loving – someone who will provide comfort to the budding pregnancy.

In a world of rising feminism, independence and free will, the notion that our hormones have this much influence on our behaviours and taste in partners may seem unsettling. Like it or not, this entire process is being governed by an historic need to survive as a human species.

The wider effect

Oestrogen and progesterone have a far wider role than governing our sexual desires. These hormones also influence our digestion, metabolism, sensory perception, sleep, breathing patterns, stress management, moods, ambitions, motivations and energy levels. In short, these hormones influence the very essence of who we are.

So, as well as governing and regulating our periods, oestrogen and progesterone also have a systemic effect on our physical and mental wellbeing. The magnitude of this is extremely new in the field of research, with scientists looking more closely at how something as seemingly benign as taking the oral contraceptive pill could have a profound influence on our behaviour. This follows as greater understanding of the strong influence our hormones have on our stress hormone levels, desires and behaviours, and thus a significant impact on how we behave.

This is really a profound revelation, the consequences of which are far reaching. It makes a lot of sense and shouldn't be so surprising when we take a step back and think about it. When children hit puberty, culturally we have come to expect that they will turn into grumpy, alien versions of the cute bambinos we once knew, before their hormones settle and they return to us as calm and caring adults. Similarly, women recognize that when hitting the menopause there is a profound change in sex drive, mood swings and even a rise in divorce rates, as this can be a pivotal time of personal interests changing.

Understanding the true impact of these hormones is crucial, as they are central to both the causes and the treatments of many period-related disorders. It is also a hugely influential factor when considering hormonal treatment options for period-related disorders (see pages 152–62 for more on this).

Hormone sensitivity

Oestrogen and progesterone's incidental effects on mood differ from person to person. For some, high progesterone can bring a beautifully calm and serene state of mind (which explains why some people feel incredibly relaxed during pregnancy). For others, high progesterone levels may increase anxiety and irritability and cause low moods.

Currently, there's no test that can determine a person's sensitivity to these hormones. However, simply being aware of their effects can be a game changer. By tracking your cycle and monitoring your mood patterns, you can begin to identify which hormonal phases trigger different emotional states.

By doing this I discovered that high progesterone doesn't bring me calm at all – for me it creates anxiety and agitation. Likewise, high oestrogen on its own tends to make me tearful and more susceptible to lower mood. Understanding these patterns in my own body helped me make informed choices about hormone therapy later in my own treatment pathways. I knew, for instance, that taking oestrogen-only HRT without balancing it with progesterone would be problematic for my mental health.

CHAPTER SUMMARY

Periods are far more than just the loss of blood each month, and this is why there's often a ripple effect when things go wrong. It is important to understand why we have periods and what they are; from this basis we can then explore what constitutes a *healthy* period and what the markers of this should be.

Key takeaways

- Periods are the physical loss of blood, endometrial tissue and vaginal secretions that we see each month, but this shedding is only a fraction of a complex process which dictates our fertility.
- As biological beings refined over millions of years to reproduce and survive, the intricate processes behind our periods are profound and deeply rooted in a survival mechanism process.
- Knowing our anatomy, such as differentiating our vulva from our vagina, and using the correct terminology is a lifesaving language that helps us communicate with healthcare professionals when things go wrong.

CHAPTER 2:
KNOW YOUR FLOW

HEALTHY VERSUS UNHEALTHY

Understanding your periods and knowing what your flow can tell you about your underlying gynaecological health is crucial to reclaiming ownership of your wellbeing. In this chapter we'll cover how to recognize a healthy period and how to spot the symptoms of gynaecological disease.

Our periods are more than just the loss of blood each month. Not only are they a marker of our fertility and availability to procreate, but the biological and physical processes involved in our cycles inform every aspect of our cells. Our mental and physical health is intricately entwined with our periods, therefore recognizing a healthy period from an unhealthy one isn't a luxury; it's potentially lifesaving.

So, before we dive deeper into the specific diseases affecting our menstrual health, let's look at the differences between a healthy period and markers of an unhealthy one.

THERE'S NO SUCH THING AS NORMAL

I recently stopped in the period-products aisle of my local supermarket and looked at the vast array of colourful items on display. As I've had a hysterectomy due to advanced endometriosis and have been menopausal for over five years, I usually walk past this section without a second glance. But this time I wanted to check if anything had changed since I last looked. I was hugely frustrated to see that there are still no warning labels relating to menstrual health on any of these products, and that the manufacturers are still using terms like 'normal flow' and 'heavy flow'.

Other health-related items such as constipation relief products often carry warnings that advise users to see a doctor if they need to use them repeatedly, as this could signal an underlying issue. Yet we've normalized heavy periods. Although the flow of a period does indeed vary from woman to woman, the broader societal dismissal and lack of clarity around what constitutes a 'normal' period is one of the first pitfalls we've created for women, even down to the language used on our sanitary products. Think of it this way: if the products we use are designed in a way that implies heavy or painful periods are normal, we risk encouraging women to ignore potential health issues. It's therefore no wonder that so many women suffer for years with symptoms that are warning signs of disease, without realizing that anything could be wrong.

With more and more social media posts claiming that heavy and painful periods are 'not normal', we've entered a state of chaos. We're getting conflicting messages left, right and centre, paving the way for what could be called a 'period-problem pandemic'. We face confusion at the very first hurdle: a society that can't define, or agree on, what a normal period is. And perhaps we need to ask whether we should even be using the word 'normal' at all.

'Normal for you'

Doctors often refer to bodily symptoms as 'normal for you'. An example being when discussing our bowel habits: for one person, one bowel movement a day is normal while for another, it might be three or four. Knowing your own personal 'normal' – your body's baseline – is essential. It's something I've tried to emphasize consistently to my patients. Developing strong self-awareness from head to toe enables you to recognize early signs of illness. And when it comes to health, early detection can be the difference between something being curable or incurable.

However – and this is a big however – for some women, period disorders begin from the onset of puberty. For example, a girl's very first period might require her to change a heavy flow pad every hour. But because of the terminology used on period product packaging, along with a longstanding social belief passed down through generations of women, she may begin her lifelong relationship with menstruation believing this is her 'normal'. In fact, this is not normal at all.

> My first period was like a scene from a horror film: debilitating pain and relentless flooding that continued throughout my teenage years until I was finally prescribed the oral contraceptive pill. I was repeatedly told this was 'my normal', and because period products were vaguely labelled 'heavy flow' without further explanation, I assumed this was just how things were.

We have a situation where one person might change a 'regular flow' pad every six hours, while another changes the same pad every hour – both assuming their experience is standard. In reality, their flow rates are drastically different but there is no guidance or additional information anywhere to tell them if this is okay or otherwise.

As with any aspect of health, recognizing the signs of disease requires first knowing what a healthy baseline is. Unfortunately, schools have historically failed to teach girls even the basic principles of menstrual and reproductive health beyond how to apply a sanitary pad or the importance of using a condom. As a result, girls enter the world of menstruation (and later, sexual health) unprepared and unequipped to understand their own bodies. For some women, by the time they realize that the periods they've been managing since age 12 are unhealthy, the damage has already been done and their fertility may be compromised.

WHAT IS A HEALTHY PERIOD?

I will never forget being taught in year six (fifth grade) by a school nurse that I should expect to lose 'an egg cupful of blood' each menstrual cycle. That really didn't seem like much and it felt almost trivial compared to all the fuss being made about how life-altering periods were supposed to be.

Fast forward two years and I was horrified to see what looked like two or three egg cups' worth of blood in just one night, while staying over at a friend's house. In that moment, I felt completely unprepared and genuinely believed I was dying. I called my friend over in a panic, shaking and convinced something was terribly wrong. She looked, laughed and said, 'No, that's normal.'

Right then and there, during my very first period, I had lost three times the amount described by the nurse as 'normal' and the very first response I received was: 'That's normal.' Later, I heard other women laugh when they recalled being told the same thing in school about the egg cupful of blood loss and the NHS website still references the same measure, with a small caveat that 'some women may experience heavier loss.' The egg cupful was a holy grail of periods, yet no one seemed to know any woman who had ever experienced this ideal phenomenon. This all reinforces the idea that 'normal' has no consistent measure, and that heavy periods are just something to be expected, silently endured and rarely questioned.

There is, therefore, no tangible, measurable or clearly communicated explanation of what a healthy period should look like. In this day and age, this is shocking. I've come to realize that women need a solid understanding of the foundations of period health before they can begin to recognize period disorders. To spot when something isn't right, you first need to understand what it looks like when it is working properly.

It's such a logical concept, yet for some reason we're not applying this in our sexual and reproductive health education. Girls are being taught about periods, but in such an inadequate and superficial way that many end up experiencing problematic periods from day one, completely unaware that what they're going through could be an early warning sign of gynaecological disease.

Get to know what's healthy for you

Girls are born with an average of one to two million eggs, technically known as oocytes, or 'eggs in waiting'. Following the onset of puberty, most girls will have settled into a regular menstrual rhythm by the age of 16 to 18 and, over the course of her reproductive years, a woman will experience approximately 450 periods before entering the menopausal phase.

From the onset of menstruation, a woman's hormones are in constant flux and her reproductive organs are continuously evolving, shedding, priming and cycling in preparation for a potential pregnancy, until the whole system eventually retires. With such a complex and ever-changing process, it is no wonder that multiple issues can arise.

Pain and heavy flow are often discussed in relation to periods, and while they are significant markers in how happy or healthy our periods are, they aren't the only ones. We need a clear, simple way to check in with ourselves each month and understand whether things are functioning as they should. By becoming more aware of our own patterns, it becomes easier to identify when something starts to drift off track. When you combine this awareness with a better understanding of what's happening beneath the surface – hormonal shifts, ovulation and endometrial changes – it becomes easier to pinpoint which hormone or phase of the cycle might be contributing to any issues.

Five key elements of a healthy period

There are five key markers of a healthy menstrual cycle that are a helpful way to maintain an overview of your menstrual health.

1. Cycle length

This refers to the number of days from the first day of your period to the first day of the next. For most people, this is around 28 days, but a healthy range is between 21 and 32 days. Ovulation – when the 'chosen' egg is released – usually occurs around the halfway point, approximately on day 14 of a 28-day cycle.

The first 14 days are spent preparing for ovulation and the following 14 days allow time for potential fertilization and implantation. If pregnancy does not occur, the body sheds the prepared uterine lining (the endometrium) and the next period begins.

2. Flow

Your flow is how heavy or light your bleeding is. Menstrual blood loss is difficult to measure accurately, but the NHS resources estimate around three to five tablespoons per cycle. Flow will vary day by day and the pattern of flow you can begin to recognize as your own natural rhythm should be consistent each month.

It's important to remember that a period is not just blood; it includes endometrial tissue, cervical mucus and vaginal secretions. A period typically starts with light spotting, then becomes heavier for two to three days before gradually tapering off. This is why early bleeding may be bright red (fresh), while later blood becomes darker brown as it ages.

It is entirely normal for flow to vary day by day over the four to seven days of menstruation. As a result, switching between lighter and heavier menstrual products throughout your period is completely reasonable. It is when this flow becomes problematic that it crosses into the realm of being 'unhealthy' (see page 67).

3. Pain

Some mild cramping or discomfort is expected during a period, as the uterus contracts to shed the endometrial lining. Using a hot water bottle or taking a warm bath is a reasonable response to a 'healthy period'.

Ovulation itself can also cause slight discomfort in some women, due to fluid released when the egg exits the ovary. Some women can even pinpoint the exact moment of ovulation and which ovary released the egg. This is a stitch-like sensation lasting a few minutes to a few hours, notably on one side. I, unfortunately, was one of them. However, while uncomfortable I did find amusement in knowing which ovary was the 'chosen' one each month.

4. The 'in-between' time

The 21 or so days between periods are often overlooked, but so much activity is happening beneath the surface and influencing our mood and physical wellbeing. While usually a 'silent' time, inter-menstrual spotting may signal an underlying problem.

Ovulation can also bring noticeable changes in vaginal discharge, such as a slight increase in quantity, a shift in colour or a temporary spotting episode. Paying attention to these subtle signs can provide insight into what's happening hormonally.

5. Mood

As discussed on pages 25–33, oestrogen and progesterone don't just influence your reproductive organs; they also affect your mood, memory and emotions.

I worry that many women are misdiagnosed with mood disorders when, in fact, they may simply be highly sensitive to hormonal fluctuations. Sadly, this can result in being prescribed antidepressants when what's really needed is a closer look at individual hormone balance.

Tracking your mood daily, weekly and monthly can help identify cyclical patterns, which may suggest a hormone-mediated cause (see page 55).

These five elements of the menstrual cycle can help women understand what is normal for them, or, more importantly, determine whether their cycle is healthy. As you'll discover on page 43, just because something has been your 'normal' since your first period doesn't necessarily mean it's healthy.

> What's considered healthy can vary from woman to woman – there's a range of acceptable values. There is no single definition of a 'healthy period' that applies to everyone, but there is a spectrum, and understanding the variations is key to understanding your own cycle.

Periods change over time

Your cycle can evolve, particularly after major life events like pregnancy or as you approach perimenopause. As you read this book and begin tuning into your own version of 'period health' (i.e. what's healthy for you), keep in mind that sudden, significant changes can signal something more serious.

For example, if someone has always had problem-free periods and then suddenly begin experiencing heavy bleeding, flooding or intense pain, it may be a sign of an underlying condition, or in rare cases a malignancy. Similarly, any bleeding that occurs after menopause (i.e. when periods have been absent for 12 months or more) is a red flag and should never be ignored.

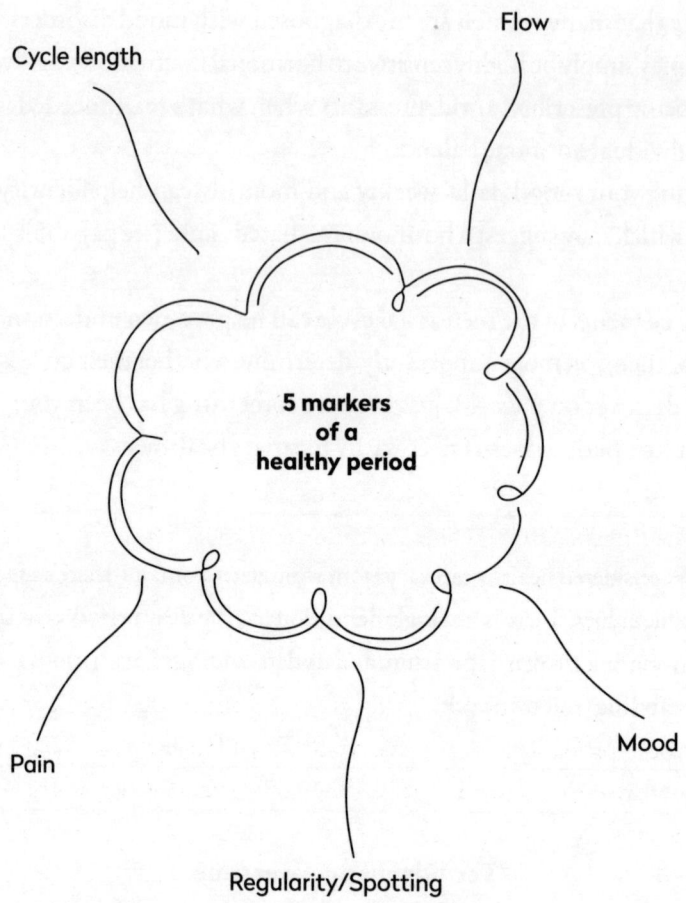

MARKERS OF AN UNHEALTHY PERIOD

Having outlined the ways in which a period *should* behave, we can now begin to explore how what we see on our sanitary products and feel in our bodies and minds might be giving us clues to the state of our gynaecological health. While there is no 'normal', the parameters for 'healthy' do exist. When one or more of these markers becomes problematic and disrupts our daily life, ability to work or thrive, we need to listen.

> Heavy and painful periods that are problematic and causing a negative impact on any part of a woman's quality of life are not healthy and should not be ignored or belittled.
>
> Pain and heavy bleeding are not healthy and can be a medical problem in themselves. While they can be the markers of more serious underlying diseases such as endometriosis (see page 73), adenomyosis (see page 201) or fibroids (see page 185), not every woman with painful or heavy periods will necessarily have an underlying cause. The existence of heavy and painful periods is – in itself – a condition that can be treated and supported, and does not need to be 'tolerated'.

Which period was 'the one'

If you're reading this book, chances are you can relate to having problematic periods of some kind. Whether you've received a diagnosis or not, you – like 90 per cent of women – may be struggling to make sense of whether your period is 'normal', or rather, healthy.

If I were to ask you to pinpoint the moment you realized your period wasn't 'normal', you'd probably look confused and stare blankly at me. That's because, culturally, we've created an environment where unhealthy periods have been so normalized that many women can no longer tell what's typical and what's not. For many of us, the answer is either, 'Probably since my very first period,' or simply, 'I'm not sure.'

While writing this book, I tried to reflect on the exact moment I realized my periods were unhealthy. Despite experiencing severely problematic periods from the very beginning (menarche), it took over 15 years before I began to acknowledge that something might be wrong. And even then, there was no formal diagnosis. There was no moment where I was told I had a gynaecological disease. No explanation of what it meant for my future, no discussion of limitations, fertility or long-term expectations. No counselling. None of the things you might expect from a consultation about a life-long, incurable condition.

All women remember their very first period. For me, that memory is now steeped in irony and despair as I reflect on how it set the tone for cultural conditioning, inadequate education and the missed opportunity to protect my fertility and organ function.

I remember girls at school hunched over in the changing rooms, doubled over with cramps. Tying jumpers around our waists in fear of visibly leaking. The sacred best-friend ritual of walking behind each other to check the back of each other's skirts for blood stains to save us from public embarrassment. Medically speaking, none of these behaviours is 'normal'; so why are they so familiar to so many of us?

Our period symptoms are a clue to the underlying cause.

AN INTRODUCTION TO PERIOD-RELATED DISORDERS

When one of the five markers of a healthy period (see page 39) falls outside the expected range, a period problem arises. Medically, this is classified as a menstrual disorder – a real, recognized condition that warrants attention and care just like any other medical diagnosis.

Awareness around pain and heavy bleeding (defined medically as blood loss exceeding 80ml/5½ tablespoons over seven days) has certainly improved, but from a clinical perspective, menstrual disorders can be broadly grouped into three key categories:

- Bleeding
- Pain
- Mood

Although women may face a range of symptoms, from headaches to bloating and insomnia to acne, as we can see in the graphic opposite, by returning to the five key markers of a healthy period, we can begin to pinpoint where the problem lies by grouping them under one of these three categories. While the 'five markers' are often used as a guide to help women group their symptoms, the conditions causing these fall into the above three categories.

KNOW YOUR FLOW

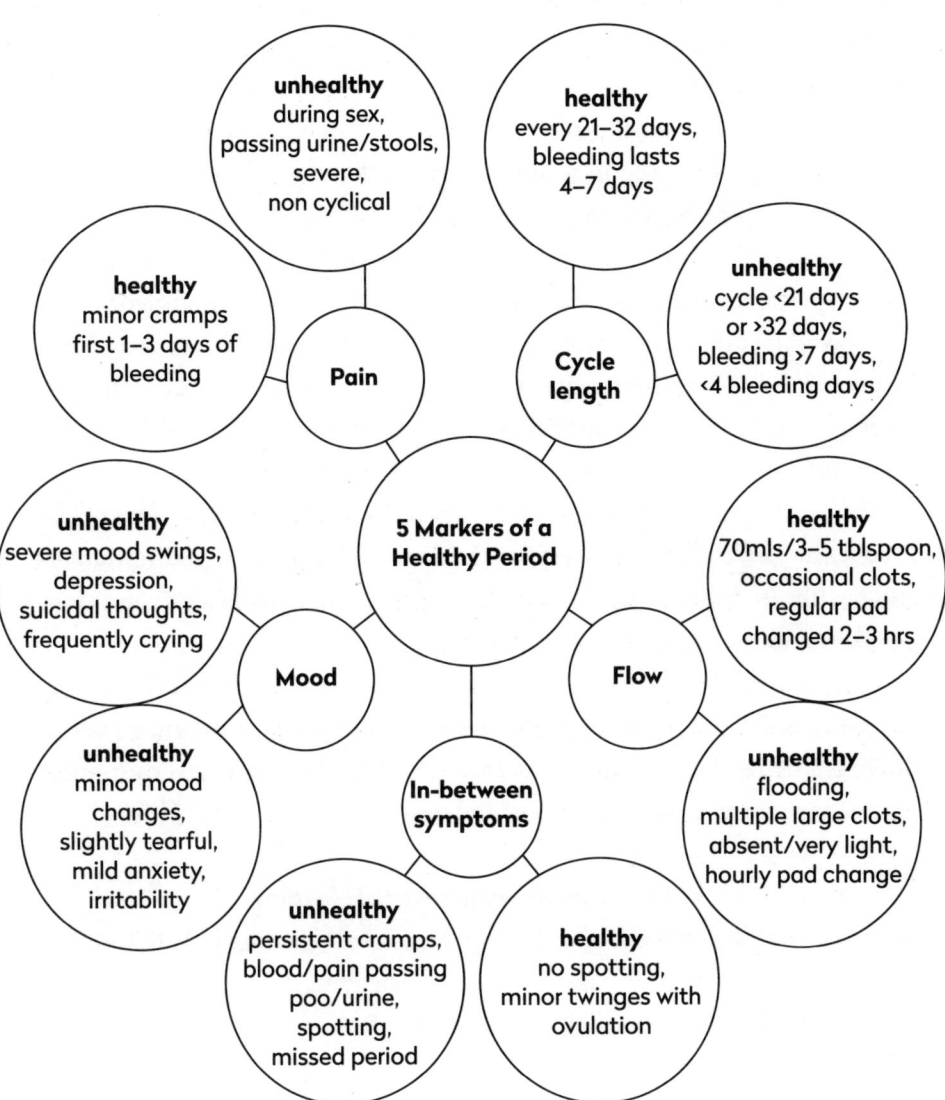

WHEN BLEEDING BECOMES A PROBLEM

At some point in history the medical reference for expected volume loss of a period was defined as '80mls'. Whoever defined heavy menstrual bleeding as 'blood loss exceeding 80ml (5½ tablespoons) within seven days' has obviously not had to stare at a used sanitary product blankly trying to figure out what this much blood looks like.

The fact that medical guidelines include an acknowledgement of the difficulties to quantitatively measure our flow speaks volumes (pun intended). To put it simply: if your bleeding feels excessive – if there's flooding, if you're doubling up on pads, leaking through clothes, feeling faint or if the bleeding lasts beyond seven days – it is entirely reasonable to label this as heavy menstrual bleeding.

Heavy bleeding is not healthy; it is a clinical concern in its own right. Moreover, heavy or problematic bleeding that a woman herself considers excessive, especially if it interrupts her quality of life physically, socially, emotionally or materially, is, in and of itself, a diagnosable issue.

This is recognized in the NICE (National Institute for Health and Care Excellence) guidelines, which serve as the national framework guiding doctors and healthcare professionals in identifying and managing health conditions based on evidence and clinical best practice.

Menorrhagia (heavy periods) are not healthy, or 'normal'. They can be severely disruptive and should not be dismissed as something women must simply endure. There is a defined clinical pathway for GPs and other clinicians to support women in managing these symptoms and regaining their quality of life.

What causes heavy menstrual bleeding

We can broadly divide women with heavy menstrual bleeding (HMB) into two groups: 50 per cent will have no identifiable underlying disease, while the other 50 per cent will have a detectable cause. But 100 per cent of these women are experiencing a real problem.

> Although the biggest symptom of fibroids is heavy bleeding (there can be pain, but the heavy bleeding is commonly the main symptom), not all women presenting with heavy bleeding will have underlying fibroids.

Dysfunctional uterine bleeding (DUB)/Primary menorrhagia

For women experiencing heavy menstrual bleeding (HMB) without a clear underlying cause, the diagnosis is often labelled in medical notes as dysfunctional uterine bleeding (DUB). In essence, this diagnosis is simply a description of the problem itself, which can feel incredibly dismissive. What's frequently not explained clearly to patients is that HMB or DUB is a recognized period-related disorder in its own right with established treatment pathways.

Even if you are told there is no underlying cause when you are experiencing heavy periods, this does not mean there is not a problem. What it really means is that there is no disease process (e.g. fibroids, endometriosis or a bleeding disorder) driving the symptoms. But the dysfunction still exists. To put it metaphorically: the orchestra is playing the right instruments, the conductor is following the correct cues, yet somehow the music just isn't coming out right. There's nothing visibly 'broken' to fix, but there are ways to manage the discord. (See page 67 for more on primary menorrhagia.)

Underlying causes/Secondary menorrhagia

Fifty per cent of women with HMB will be told that this is due to one (or a combination) of the following:

- Fibroids (see page 185)
- Adenomyosis (see page 201)
- Endometriosis (see page 73)
- Uterine cancer
- Systemic problems (e.g. coagulation disorders, thyroid diseases)
- IUD (intrauterine device, commonly called the coil)
- Medications such as anticoagulants

Other bleeding-related period disorders

Blood loss with periods is not simply a case of heavy or not; erratic, irregular, spotting or too light are also markers of underlying problems. The table on page 49 outlines the various bleeding-related issues that can arise and what might cause them.

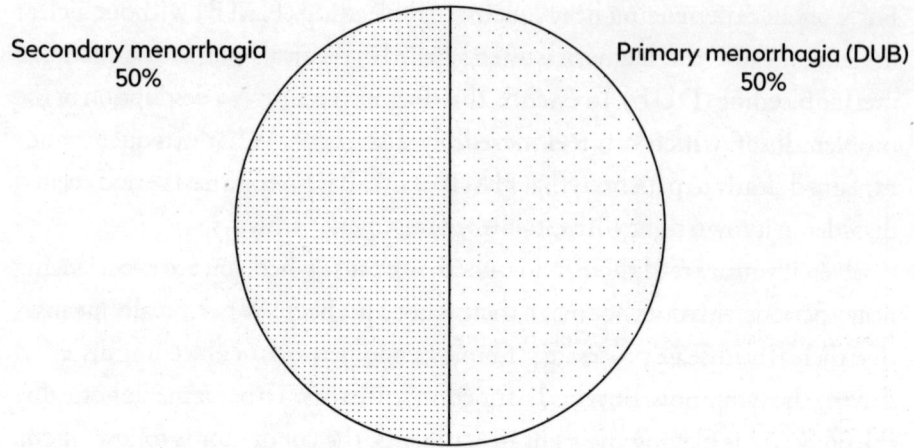

Percentage of women experiencing heavy periods: 50 per cent will have primary menorrhagia and 50 per cent will have a secondary cause.

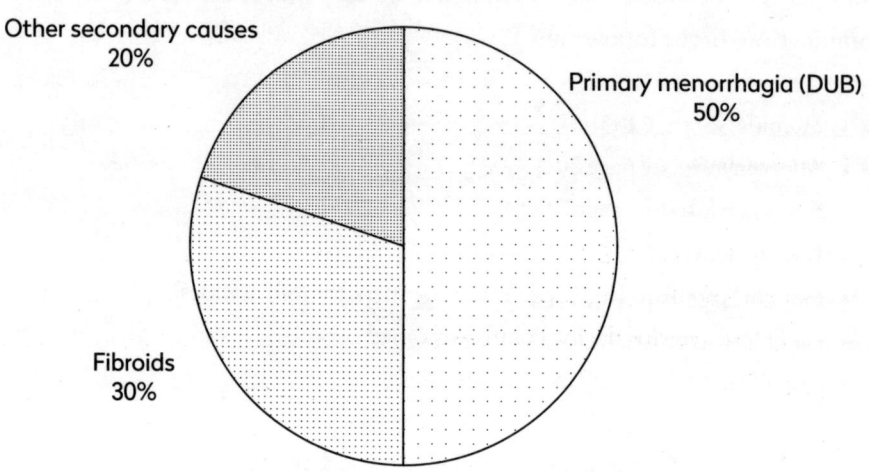

Fibroids is the cause for approximately a third of women complaining of heavy periods.

Condition	Bleeding Pattern	Underlying Causes
Menorrhagia	Heavy/excessive bleeding > 80mls (5½ tbsp) > 7 days	Fibroids Uterine cancer Endometriosis Adenomyosis Systemic conditions (e.g. coagulation disorders, thyroid disease) Medications
Metrorrhagia	Irregular bleeding	PCOS (polycystic ovary syndrome)
Oligomenorrhoea	Infrequent bleeding	PCOS (polycystic ovary syndrome) Endocrine disorders Weight problems
Amenorrhoea	Absence of periods	Primary infertility Primary ovulatory insufficiency PCOS (polycystic ovary syndrome) Malignancy Endocrine disorders Anorexia
Hypomenorrhoea	Lighter than expected	

PAINFUL PERIODS/DYSMENORRHOEA

Dysmenorrhoea is perhaps the most misunderstood of all the period-related disorders, possibly even more so than fibroids (see page 185) or heavy bleeding (see page 67).

> 50 per cent of women who experience heavy menstrual bleeding won't be diagnosed with an underlying cause (they will have primary menorrhagia). This jumps to 90 per cent of women who have painful periods.

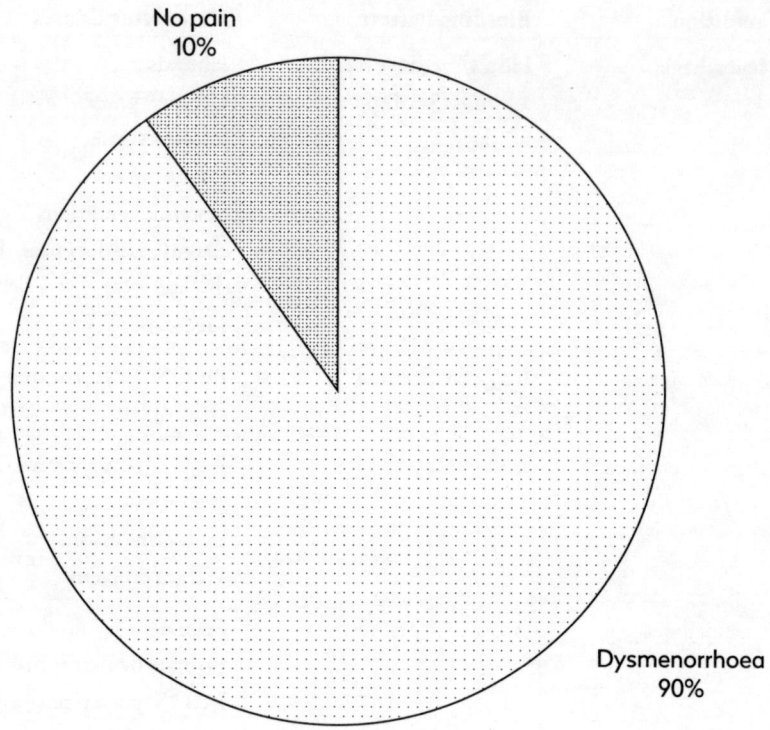

90 per cent of women will seek medical attention for painful periods (dysmenorrhoea) during their reproductive years.

Primary dysmenorrhoea

Primary dysmenorrhoea is where the cause of the pain is due to the process of menstruation itself, rather than due to a secondary disease such as endometriosis (see page 73). The absence of a secondary cause does not mean that painful periods are 'normal' just because they are the result of a physiological process. They are an over-reaction, a dysfunction and a very real problem for many women, with equally real options for support.

Pain, in almost every other context, is our body's alarm system alerting our brain (both consciously and subconsciously) that something might be wrong. It's

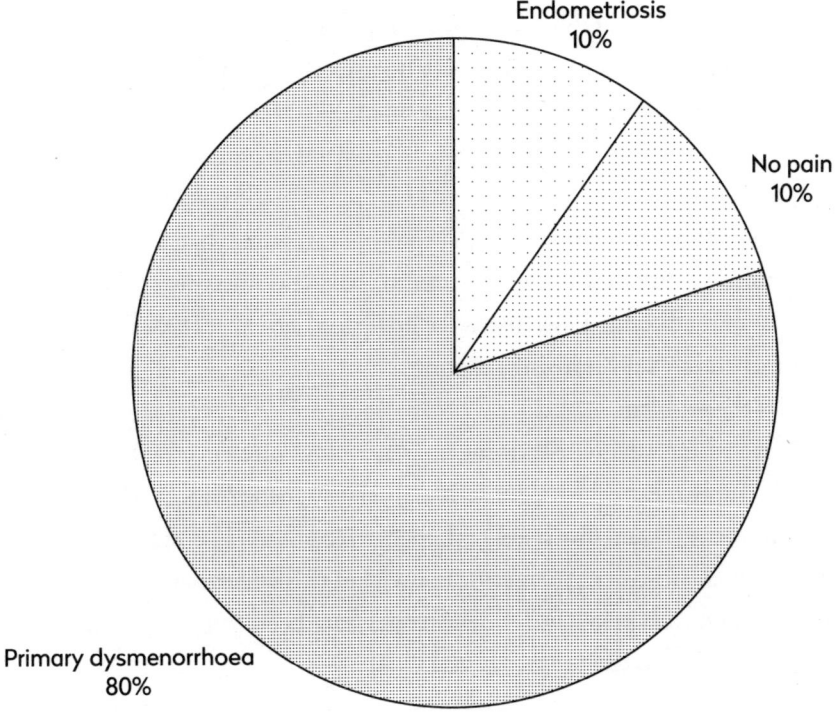

Endometriosis affects 10 per cent of women, meaning the majority of women with painful periods will have primary dysmenorrhoea.

a signal of potential danger, a threat to our wellbeing, and we're programmed to listen to it.

And that programming runs deep. Pain is almost impossible to ignore and we are hard-wired to pay attention to it. Its detection triggers a stress response in the brain to the body, including the release of cortisol to prepare us for 'fight or flight'. From an evolutionary perspective, ignoring pain could mean death.

So, when we consider that up to 90 per cent of women of reproductive age experience problematic period pain at some point – and that 90 per cent of those cases are classed as primary dysmenorrhoea (meaning without an underlying cause) – there seems to be a disconnect. But 'no underlying cause' doesn't mean there isn't a real and valid problem. Human beings (understandably) don't like being told there's no cause for their symptoms, especially when those symptoms involve pain.

There is an unfortunate common situation that can arise when a scan result or investigation determines that a woman doesn't have endometriosis or another of the familiar named conditions. Instead of being told 'no cause found' they are sometimes incorrectly told 'nothing is wrong'.

And *that's* the problem.

Clinicians without adequate training in gynaecology often overlook that 'no cause found' simply means the diagnosis is primary dysmenorrhoea rather than secondary dysmenorrhoea. Both are real, recognized medical conditions and both follow similar treatment pathways. Yet, within this wider 'period problem pandemic', women with primary dysmenorrhoea have been consistently under-supported and invalidated.

Dysmenorrhoea is divided into two categories:

Primary dysmenorrhoea: No identifiable organic cause. The pain stems from the menstrual process itself.

Secondary dysmenorrhoea: Pain caused by an underlying disease process (e.g. endometriosis, adenomyosis, fibroids) or anatomical abnormality.

'No underlying cause found'

Many women believe that the number one cause of painful periods is likely to be endometriosis, and the risk of missing a diagnosis of endometriosis can have severe implications for the preservation of a woman's gynaecological organs, quality of life and fertility. However, the majority of women with painful periods don't have endometriosis. Remember that 90 per cent of women experience painful periods, but only 10 per cent have endometriosis. This is where the confusion arises, and many women are left feeling unsupported, particularly if they have heard that their scan or surgery showed 'no underlying cause found'.

'No underlying cause found' is a medical term that simply means there is nothing structurally wrong to be seen, and no organic disease process happening that can be identified. What this does not mean is that there is nothing wrong. In this situation (no diagnosis such as endometriosis) it suggests that the actual cause for the pain is what doctors call primary dysmenorrhoea. While this has 'no obvious underlying cause' this does not mean the pain or problem does not exist. As human beings, we instinctively seek reasons; something tangible, visible or explainable. It's difficult for us to accept that something 'just is'. That's why a diagnosis of primary dysmenorrhoea, with no underlying structural cause found, can feel dismissive.

However, given that many women presenting with painful periods will not have an identifiable disease, this is precisely why not every woman is immediately referred for further investigation or surgery. What many understandably perceive as being dismissed is, in part, a clinically reasonable response to statistical probability. (See page 65 for more on managing primary dysmenorrhoea.)

SECONDARY DYSMENORRHOEA

For the 10 per cent of women experiencing painful periods who are diagnosed with secondary dysmenorrhoea following the correct investigations, the most common culprit is endometriosis. However, there are other causes and the most common are:

- Endometriosis (see page 73)
- Adenomyosis (see page 201)
- Fibroids (see page 185)

- Pelvic inflammatory disease
- IUD (intrauterine device, commonly called the coil)
- Ectopic pregnancy

These are conditions in which structural changes or disease processes disrupt the natural harmony of the reproductive organs, leading to pain and often other symptoms such as heavy bleeding, bowel cramps, pain during sex, etc.

The reason these underlying diseases have received so much attention recently is because they can be utterly devastating and permanently life-altering. Endometriosis has the potential to damage multiple organs, cause infertility and lead to a life dominated by hospital appointments, surgeries, scarring, adhesions and, in severe cases, even the formation of stomas. So, the fear of having an underlying condition missed or overlooked is completely justified.

But how is a woman supposed to know the difference between primary dysmenorrhoea and pain caused by an underlying condition like endometriosis without adequate testing? Unfortunately, there is no simple test, and because most women who present with period pain do not have endometriosis, there is also no quick or definitive way to make that distinction at the outset.

What's important to understand, however, is that the treatment options for both primary and secondary dysmenorrhoea are often very similar. In fact, the treatments available directly from a GP are often the same, whether the underlying cause is primary dysmenorrhoea or early-stage endometriosis. So, what may be perceived as a 'watch and wait' approach is not passive – it's a measured, medically sound strategy, rooted in evidence-based practice.

Whether you're being treated for primary or secondary dysmenorrhoea, the pathway your GP should follow – according to NICE guidelines – is largely the same, regardless of the underlying cause. That means the urgency for an immediate answer isn't always clinically necessary.

Is that frustrating? Absolutely.

But part of that frustration stems from the historical trivialization of painful or heavy periods. With the right support and understanding, women can feel empowered to allow time, follow the appropriate care pathway and know they are not being dismissed, but rather medically supported in a way that balances safety, evidence and sustainability.

MOOD-RELATED PROBLEMS

As with many mental health topics, acknowledging or validating something that affects our mood can be far more uncomfortable than discussing physical symptoms. If talking about menstrual flow already feels like TMI, then admitting you feel suicidal once a month definitely qualifies as oversharing.

As we discovered on page 30, oestrogen and progesterone influence not just our reproductive organs and menstrual cycle, but also our emotions and behaviours. They are the silent influencers we carry with us, often without even realizing.

Oestrogen plays a physical and behavioural role in preparing us to appear fertile and increasing libido. It gives us energy, ambition, focus and a drive to engage, encouraging us, biologically, to mate during the fertile window. Once ovulation passes and the egg is not fertilized, oestrogen steps back, making room for progesterone.

Progesterone, the so-called nesting hormone, shifts our body into preparation mode, priming the uterus for a potential pregnancy. Its influence is calming, sedative even. It promotes rest, stillness and often those familiar cravings for carbs and comfort. It doesn't want us to do anything risky that could threaten a potential embryo.

This hormonal contrast creates two very different versions of us within a single month, which is why so many women notice fluctuations in mood, motivation and energy levels. One week you're smashing it at work, bossing the gym and a sex goddess in the bedroom. The next week it's Netflix and chill, chocolate and a desperate need for a blanket and zero interaction.

But progesterone is not always the calming, zen-inducing hormone it's meant to be. Instead, it can induce crippling anxiety and depression. Similarly, oestrogen doesn't always bring confidence or libido – it can trigger internal chaos and explosive rage.

Premenstrual syndrome/tension (PMS/PMT)

The emotional and physical symptoms caused by these hormonal fluctuations are commonly referred to as PMS (premenstrual syndrome) or PMT (premenstrual tension). Some women are fortunate to experience minimal disruption, sailing through the cycle with little turbulence. But 60–80 per cent of women will experience PMS at some point during their reproductive years, and it's anything but smooth. The seatbelt sign is flashing, and you can't ignore the emotional turbulence. Progesterone doesn't just make you sleepy and snacky, it can leave you a tearful, anxious, bloated, emotionally fragile mess. That favourite dress doesn't fit, and suddenly you're spiralling into a wave of tears and self-loathing.

And just as our hormone levels shift, our symptoms can also evolve with life stages. During the teenage years, when the body is still 'finding its rhythm', fluctuations can be more extreme (especially noticeable to parents and siblings). Post-pregnancy, the hormonal equilibrium we had adapted to for years can collapse. For some women, things settle after a while. For others, the body never fully returns to its pre-pregnancy baseline.

In general practice, I met many women in their early thirties who had never struggled with PMS until they had children. After one or two pregnancies, they found themselves hit with waves of rage, visceral anger, extreme fatigue or unpredictable mood swings. The relief they felt when I reassured them that this was a common experience at their stage of reproductive life was profound. Once we acknowledged what they were going through, we could explore the options available to support them and, most importantly, help them feel seen and understood.

Premenstrual dysphoric disorder (PMDD)

If PMS is turbulence prompting the seatbelt sign to switch on, then PMDD is the oxygen masks dropping and a call to brace for impact. The stigma around mental health is already isolating and for PMDD, a condition still so poorly understood, this isolation is often magnified. Only now are we beginning to see a rise in awareness that PMDD even exists.

PMDD is PMS on a whole other level. It involves extreme, cyclical mood shifts, where one week a woman may feel calm, in control and thriving in her life, work and relationships, and just a few days later that same woman may feel suicidal, consumed by rage, despair and intrusive thoughts. Alongside these emotional changes, PMDD often includes physical symptoms: headaches, muscle aches, bloating, insomnia or intense lethargy that makes getting out of bed feel impossible.

The science hasn't fully pinpointed the cellular cause of PMDD, but the current scientific theory suggests it's not that women with PMDD produce too much of any hormone. Instead, their brains and hormone receptors are hypersensitive, triggering an exaggerated response to normal hormonal fluctuations.

Centuries of misogyny and medical gaslighting – with archaic phrases like 'female hysteria' – have contributed to the dangerous misconception that these reactions are within a woman's control. They are not. PMDD is a real physiological condition where the body is having an abnormal response to a 'normal' menstrual cycle process.

As understanding of PMDD grows through advancing research, I wouldn't be surprised if some women come to realize their bipolar diagnosis was a misdiagnosis. Not out of negligence, but because the profound impact of hormones on mental health is only now starting to be fully appreciated.

Postnatal mood disorders

This hypersensitivity to hormones is what lies behind the postnatal emotional storm for some women – baby blues, postnatal depression, even postnatal psychosis. If I had known all this earlier in life, I would have been far more vigilant for postnatal depression. In my case, progesterone triggers overwhelming anxiety and low mood. During the postnatal period, when the body floods with calming hormones to encourage lactation, I spiralled into a postnatal depression so severe I didn't even recognize myself, let alone my own thoughts.

Understanding how your hormones affect your mood

All women are unique, and it can take time to understand ourselves and our cycles. There's no predictability to these responses but tracking your cycle and building awareness of your individual patterns can be hugely empowering.

For women unaware of just how powerfully hormones can affect mood, drive and motivation, these erratic shifts and intrusive thoughts can feel terrifying. The fear of judgement, of being labelled or misunderstood – whether by society or by healthcare professionals – keeps so many women from seeking the help they need. But imagine the relief of realizing that hormonal support could ease or even eliminate those thoughts? That these overwhelming emotions weren't a character flaw or mental illness, but a misfiring hormonal response?

That's why, for me, menopause was a welcome relief – not just from the physical pain of endometriosis, but from the havoc of hormonal swings. The stability of mood, the disappearance of anxiety and the steady, consistent mental state far outweighed any inconvenience of hot flushes or being menopausal in my early thirties.

While there's absolutely a valid role for antidepressants, there are also many women who present with mood-related symptoms that are, in fact, the result of hormonal hypersensitivity, not a primary mental health condition. The exciting thing is that research is finally catching up, and we're beginning to shine a light on the intricate relationship between hormones and mood.

CHAPTER SUMMARY

The wonderfully delightful detail to add to everything above is this: many women don't just experience one period-related problem (why would Mother Nature be so kind, after all?). For most women, these conditions and symptoms overlap and can present so gradually that they became 'normal for us' and we don't realize that our periods are providing us with clues as to our underlying health status.

Unfortunately, many secondary causes of dysmenorrhoea and menorrhagia, such as endometriosis and adenomyosis, are rarely limited to painful or heavy periods. Instead, they often bring the full package: headaches, bloating, fatigue, mood swings and more. And if the body is already under stress from such underlying conditions, there's often an added layer of hormonal sensitivity, meaning the emotional turbulence is thrown in for good measure. So, we're rarely dealing with just one symptom, like pain or flooding. We're talking about a complex, whole-body experience that affects us physically, mentally and emotionally.

But here's the good news: understanding all of this – really breaking down the conditions and how they affect you – can be genuinely empowering. It gives

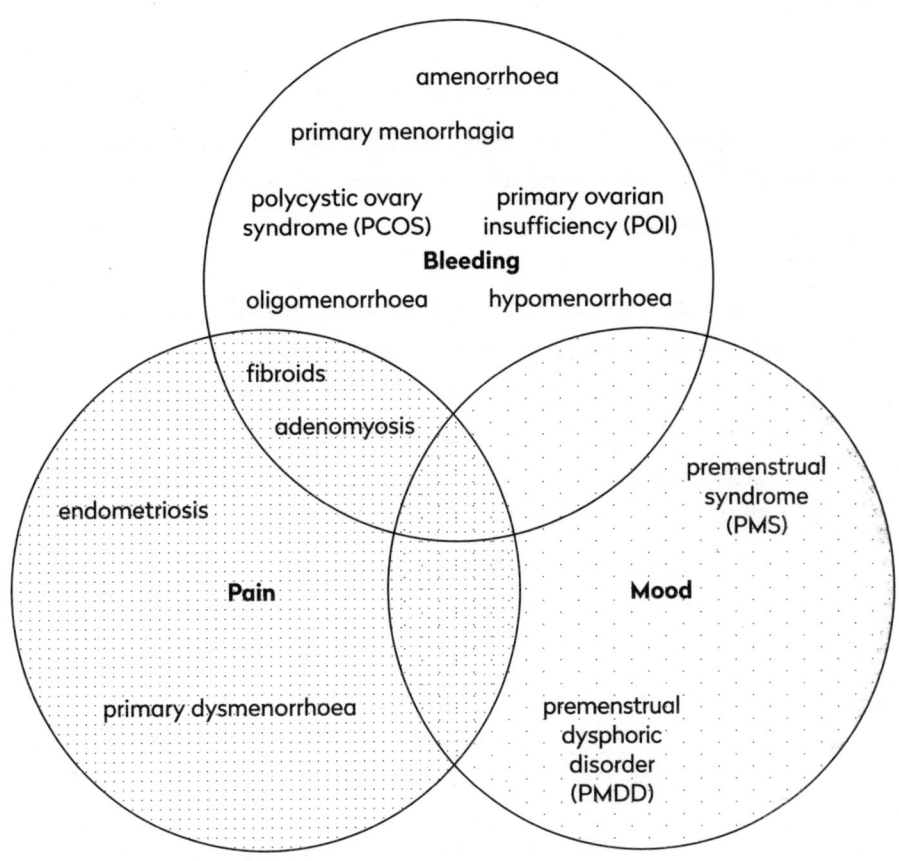

Conditions categorized into main presenting symptom

you the tools to regain a sense of control over your body (and sometimes even your sanity).

I always tell patients, and anyone who asks me for advice, that understanding the mental and emotional implications of these conditions – and their treatments – is just as important as understanding the physical aspects. They are not separate entities. Recognizing the connection between hormones, symptoms and emotional wellbeing opens an entirely new level of self-awareness. Whether you have a good or difficult relationship with certain hormones, having this knowledge gives you more autonomy and confidence in choosing the right treatment options for you.

Key takeaways

- A healthy period is one which should not impact on your quality of life or ability to thrive. If symptoms are significant enough to cause impact, then a diagnosis should be sought, and as with any diagnosis there are options for treatment or support.
- For the majority of women who experience painful periods (dysmenorrhoea) and heavy bleeding (menorrhagia), there is no underling disease and problems arise from a dysfunction within the process of menstruation itself. Just because no cause (in terms of a secondary disease process) is found, does not mean that no problem exists – and support is available.
- Secondary causes of dysmenorrhoea and menorrhagia are less common (e.g. endometriosis or fibroids) and sometimes hard to diagnose, but treatment can begin while looking for the answers. The treatments for both primary and secondary overlap which means 'trusting the process' – and beginning treatment while waiting for answers is a process that can be trusted.

CHAPTER 3:
PRIMARY DYSMENORRHOEA AND PRIMARY MENORRHAGIA

NO UNDERLYING CAUSE DOES NOT MEAN NO PROBLEM

Primary dysmenorrhoea (painful periods) and **primary menorrhagia** (heavy periods) are caused when the process of menstruation itself behaves in a dysfunctional way. When there is a disease process at work, such as endometriosis or fibroids, this is known as **secondary dysmenorrhoea** or **menorrhagia**.

Whether primary or secondary, the impact of these disrupting your quality of life remains equally deserving of answers. Both deserve understanding of what is happening, and what management is available to help. The process of diagnosing primary dysmenorrhoea (PD) or primary menorrhagia (PM) is one of exclusion, which can take time. During that time, your doctor will begin treatments (often hormone based) to manage/improve your symptoms. These initial hormone treatments that target pain and regulate periods overlap for many of the potential underlying causes, which is why you can be reassured that although the wait for a definitive answer can feel prolonged, this wait is not without support.

A woman can potentially wait several years as investigations are carried out and treatments trialled; during this time, she may expect an underlying diagnosis of endometriosis only to be told there is no secondary organic cause. Unfortunately, this isn't always followed with adequate communication to explain that the absence of a secondary cause does not mean there is no diagnosis. This lack of understanding means that so many women aren't getting the treatment they need and deserve. Remember: no woman should be left feeling their heavy and painful periods are normal or that there is no hope of regaining a healthy period.

PRIMARY DYSMENORRHOEA (PD)

Ninety per cent of women will experience dysmenorrhoea (painful periods) during their reproductive years, but the majority of them will have 'no underlying cause'. But there is scientific proof that PD is very real indeed, and there is a physiological process behind it.

What is period pain?

I recently came across a social media video comparing period pain to a heart attack, and I'll be honest, I wanted to bang my head against the desk. I was aghast. While I understand the logic behind it (clickbait meets good intentions), it's yet another example of facts being twisted for shock value. And while that might generate likes, it creates unnecessary panic and confusion – neither of which we need more of in women's health.

It's important to adequately understand what's happening when we experience period pain. Pain (in general terms) is a deeply primal phenomenon, a signal to the brain that something might threaten our safety or health. It triggers a cascade of hormonal and stress responses, including the release of cortisol, because we are biologically wired not to ignore pain. When you're in pain, you don't just want it numbed – you want to know why it's happening so you can feel reassured that nothing sinister is being overlooked.

So, let's go deep inside those uterine muscle cells and nerve pathways for a moment and explore what's going on within the uterus to manifest such pain.

The science (made human)

When we talk about period pain, we're really talking about the activity of a group of chemical messengers known as prostaglandins.

Think of prostaglandins as the body's dispatchers – they send rapid instructions to different tissues to respond to injury, infection or change. Like hormones, they communicate with the body, telling blood to clot, blood vessels to constrict or dilate and inflammatory responses to activate when something needs healing. Prostaglandins are created through a chain of events involving enzymes called COX enzymes (short for cyclooxygenase). These enzymes help trigger the production of prostaglandins when the body detects change or stress.

In the heart, for example, prostaglandins are released when blood flow is blocked by a clot, which contributes to the pain of a heart attack (ischaemia). So yes, period pain and heart attack pain share a similar mechanism – at a *chemical level* – but let's be clear: a heart attack is life-threatening, and period pain is not.

So, what causes the pain? Every month, the endometrial lining builds up under the influence of oestrogen and progesterone, ready to receive a fertilized egg. When pregnancy doesn't happen, hormone levels drop suddenly. That hormonal drop triggers a biological chain reaction: COX enzymes activate, prostaglandins surge and the uterus receives its monthly 'instruction' to contract.

Those contractions serve a purpose: they constrict the blood vessels in the uterine wall, cutting off blood flow just enough to help the lining shed and reset the menstrual cycle. It's a perfectly natural process – a controlled, temporary mini-storm in the uterus.

The result for most women is mild cramping: a gentle reminder of the cycle turning over. Some barely notice it. But for others, the contractions are stronger, the prostaglandin levels higher and the sensitivity to pain receptors heightened – known as primary dysmenorrhoea.

When things go wrong

In primary dysmenorrhoea, everything is technically 'working' – it's just working too hard. The uterus produces too many prostaglandins, the contractions become too intense and the temporary reduction in blood flow becomes more pronounced. Add to that the fact that some women have nerve receptors that are hypersensitive to pain (often influenced by oestrogen), and the pain signals sent to the brain can be amplified far beyond what's needed.

This isn't psychological and it's not weakness or a symptom of having a low pain threshold. It's quite the opposite, in fact; it's a biological overreaction. The nerves and chemical messengers are simply overzealous, turning up the volume far louder than the body needs.

And because there's a real, measurable mechanism behind it, there are also real, effective treatments. That's the silver lining here. Most women with primary dysmenorrhoea can be well supported through GP-led care without needing specialist referral.

Seeking a diagnosis

How do you tell the difference between primary dysmenorrhoea (PD) and one of the secondary causes such as endometriosis or adenomyosis (see pages 73 and 201)? I can almost hear the mental checklists forming as women everywhere start reviewing their own symptoms.

In medicine, diagnosis is often a process of detective work. Doctors piece together patterns, timings and clusters of symptoms, always keeping context in mind about your age, your history and your overall health.

Primary dysmenorrhoea typically begins in the teenage years, once periods become established. Those underlying mechanisms of hypersensitive nerves and overenthusiastic prostaglandin production often show themselves early, becoming the 'default setting' of your cycle.

The pain pattern of PD follows a fairly recognizable script:

- The pain usually starts just before the period begins.
- It lasts for the first few days of bleeding.
- It subsides as the flow lightens.
- And crucially, it isn't accompanied by other 'red flag' symptoms (see below).

If you have pain mid-cycle or during or after sex, bleeding between periods or bowel and bladder symptoms, those are clues that something else might be at play, likely one of the secondary causes.

PD, on the other hand, tends to be predictable. The pain comes, it goes, and it follows the rhythm of your cycle. Secondary causes often appear later, usually in your twenties or thirties, although they can, of course, show up earlier.

This is why keeping a symptom diary is so valuable. When you walk into your GP appointment able to answer yes/no to those 'other symptom' questions, you're giving them a map straight to the right diagnosis.

If your symptoms fit the typical pattern of PD, your GP will likely start with treatment straight away. If there's any doubt, they may request an ultrasound, MRI or other investigations, not to delay you, but to rule out those secondary causes while also starting treatment in parallel. And that's key: you don't have to wait for a final diagnosis to begin relief.

Management

While there's no cure for primary dysmenorrhoea, because technically there's nothing structurally wrong to fix – the system is functioning, it's just overreacting – there are treatment options.

If we consider the menstrual cycle as an orchestra, in PD the conductor isn't missing, she's just wildly overenthusiastic. The right instruments are in place, the melody is correct, but the music is painfully loud. The solution isn't to fire the orchestra, it's to calm it down.

Non-hormonal options

Paracetamol can certainly help with general discomfort, and the group of analgesics we know as NSAIDs (non-steroidal anti-inflammatories) are far better suited to PD pain. This is because the real culprits of the pain are prostaglandins, and NSAIDs such as ibuprofen specifically inhibit the chemical process that produces prostaglandins, reducing the intensity of contractions and easing pain at its root. (Please note that NSAIDs are best taken with food to protect the stomach; they are not suitable in pregnancy or suspected pregnancy.)

Many women assume paracetamol and ibuprofen are interchangeable but they're not. If paracetamol hasn't worked for you, it doesn't mean nothing will. Regular, timed use of ibuprofen or naproxen in the first few days of your period can make a world of difference.

There's also a group of medications called COX inhibitors which directly block the enzymes that create prostaglandins. These are especially helpful for women who can't tolerate NSAIDs and can be prescribed by your GP.

Hormonal options

The contraceptive pill (whether combined oestrogen–progesterone or progesterone-only) can essentially 'override' the menstrual cycle. The bleed that occurs while on hormonal contraceptives is a 'pseudo-period'. With no ovulation occurring, there's minimal endometrial build-up and therefore fewer prostaglandins. By calming the entire hormonal rhythm, these options can dramatically reduce both pain and heavy bleeding. Speak to your GP to see if the contraceptive pill might be suitable for you.

Non-medical approaches

I am a huge advocate for recognizing that sometimes the simple tools do genuinely help:

- Heat (for example, a covered hot-water bottle or heat pad) placed over the lower stomach can help by dilating the blood vessels, which improves blood flow to cramping muscles.
- Warm baths work by the same mechanism as above, plus they offer relaxation.
- Exercise improves circulation, releases endorphins and reduces inflammation.
- TENS machines provide targeted pain relief.

Finding the right combination of support can take time. Remember, you only get one cycle a month to test new treatments, so patience is part of the process. If something stops working or new symptoms arise that don't fit the pattern of PD, that's your cue to go back to your GP and reassess.

Because yes, there can be overlap. Someone who had PD in her teens could develop endometriosis or adenomyosis later in life. This doesn't necessarily indicate a 'missed' diagnosis; sometimes circumstances change. Knowing your cycle and what is your normal is essential for spotting if something new develops.

A teenager started on the contraceptive pill at 18 for painful periods (that worked) and later diagnosed with endometriosis at 28 hasn't necessarily been 'ignored' for a decade, as the disease may have developed over time.

I say this to rebuild trust where it's been understandably shaken: most GPs are doing their best with imperfect tools. The key is persistence, communication and collaboration. If something isn't working or it used to work but doesn't anymore, revisit the plan.

PRIMARY MENORRHAGIA (PM)

Primary menorrhagia (PM) is where heavy, excessive bleeding is *not* due to an underlying disease such as fibroids. Around half of all women who present with heavy bleeding fall into the category of primary menorrhagia. In simple terms, it is dysfunctional uterine bleeding without an obvious or organic cause.

What causes heavy bleeding?

The answer mirrors that of primary dysmenorrhoea (see page 62). Everything in the menstrual orchestra is technically in place, all the musicians are there reading the right notes, but the tempo is off. If primary dysmenorrhoea is the orchestra playing too loudly, primary menorrhagia is the orchestra playing too fast.

With PM, the issue is often that one or more of the regulatory systems within menstruation is slightly overactive.

- The endometrium (lining of the uterus) may be overstimulated by hormones, thickening more than necessary.
- Prostaglandins and other chemical messengers might be overproduced or imbalanced, influencing blood vessel constriction and clotting in a way that increases blood loss.
- The clotting process itself might not quite kick in effectively enough to slow the flow.

The outcome is the same: heavy, prolonged and often unpredictable bleeding, sometimes accompanied by cramps, fatigue or anaemia. Primary menorrhagia can happen at any age, and the natural shifts that come with pregnancy, birth or perimenopause can all change how your uterus behaves.

It's crucial to first rule out the secondary causes because these can look similar but require different treatments. Once secondary causes are ruled out, primary menorrhagia becomes a diagnosis in its own right. This is not a dismissal, not a dead end, but a recognized condition with its own evidence-based treatments. Unfortunately, the reality is that women are often told 'there are no fibroids or signs of disease' and not told that their heavy bleeding still warrants a diagnosis and, more importantly, has options for support.

Seeking a diagnosis

Primary menorrhagia is one of those curious medical diagnoses where the answer is found not by discovering what's wrong, but by confirming what's not.

Your GP will begin by taking a detailed history: what your periods are like, how long they last, how often you change sanitary products and whether you experience clots, pain or fatigue. They'll likely perform an examination and consider simple investigations such as:

- Blood tests to check for anaemia or clotting disorders.
- Ultrasound scans to look for fibroids, polyps or uterine thickening.
- Possibly a hysteroscopy, where a tiny camera checks the lining of the uterus.

All of this can be arranged through your GP, with no referral needed initially. If none of these tests reveals a clear culprit and your history fits the picture, then the diagnosis of primary menorrhagia will be made. It's not a diagnosis of exclusion in the dismissive sense; it's a diagnosis of dysfunction where the system is doing too much of what it's supposed to do.

Many women are put on the contraceptive pill for this exact reason but totally unaware that this is their underlying diagnosis. This mismatch goes back to the need for open communication between GP and patient. Realizing your hormonal contraceptives are being used to manage a period disorder gives you the awareness to become even more in tune with your body so you can monitor for other red flags that may later arise and indicate a need to revisit the diagnosis. When something changes in your symptoms then the diagnosis may need to be reviewed.

Management

The good news is that while investigations are ongoing, you don't have to sit in limbo without help. The first-line treatments for heavy bleeding regardless of cause include:

- **NSAIDs** (non-steroidal anti-inflammatory drugs) such as ibuprofen or naproxen: not only for pain but because they also reduce prostaglandin levels, which helps lessen bleeding.
- **Tranexamic acid**: a medication that helps blood clot more effectively within the uterus, reducing blood loss.
- **Hormonal treatments**: such as the combined pill, progesterone-only pill or IUS (intrauterine system, commonly called the hormonal coil), which thin the endometrial lining and significantly reduce bleeding over time.

These are often started by the GP while further tests are arranged. This is not delaying care, it's proactive management. It means you're being treated while your body's unique version of the menstrual orchestra is being studied in more detail.

It's completely understandable to feel anxious or frustrated when there's no neat label attached to your symptoms, but rest assured, lack of a secondary cause does not mean lack of support. Your quality of life still matters and you are still amenable to, and entitled to, treatment to provide relief from the burdensome flooding.

CHAPTER SUMMARY

I often speak with women who feel utterly deflated, even betrayed, after years of seeking answers for their painful or heavy periods. They've fought tooth and nail for a diagnosis, finally reached the point of getting a laparoscopy, only to be told: 'We found nothing.' For one woman I spoke to, that moment was devastating. She had pinned her hopes on being told she had endometriosis, not because she wanted a disease, but because she wanted validation. Instead, she left the hospital in tears – still in pain, still bleeding heavily and now with no clear direction. That reaction is understandable. It's not just about the physical symptoms, it's about being seen, believed and reassured that what you're experiencing isn't being dismissed.

It's crucial to understand that the absence of a secondary cause does not mean there's nothing wrong. It simply means the cause is primary; a dysfunction of the menstrual system itself. And dysfunctions can be treated, supported and improved.

Both primary dysmenorrhoea and primary menorrhagia are legitimate medical conditions. They are not lesser diagnoses and they are not figments of imagination. They're the body's systems slightly over-performing – the orchestra playing too loudly or too fast – and they can absolutely be managed.

When these primary causes are correctly recognized and supported, they should not impact fertility. If infertility becomes a concern, meaning difficulty conceiving after a year of trying or recurrent miscarriages, that's a sign to revisit the diagnosis because it could suggest an underlying secondary condition.

And as always, if new symptoms appear or if a treatment stops working, it's time to go back to your GP and reopen the discussion. Period health is dynamic. What's true at 18 might not be true at 30. Your body evolves, and so should your care.

Remember that the process can take time. A menstrual cycle is only once a month, meaning every new treatment or observation takes weeks to assess. This can feel slow and frustrating, especially when you're the one living through it. But slow progress is still progress and each cycle gives more insight into your unique pattern. Keeping a symptom diary remains one of the most powerful tools you can use. Record what happens, when it happens, what helps and what doesn't. Those notes can cut months off the diagnostic process and give you tangible proof of what you're experiencing.

A healthy period should fit into your life, not dictate it. If it's interrupting your work, your plans, your sleep or your sense of normalcy, that's your body waving a flag, not because it's failing you but because it's asking for support. And support exists. You just need to know how to ask for it – and now, you do.

Key takeaways

- **Primary dysmenorrhoea** (PD) and **primary menorrhagia** are the presence of problematic pain and heavy bleeding that are beyond what should be considered 'normal' but not caused by underlying organic disease processes. These are common problems and account for a large proportion of period-related issues.
- 'No underlying cause' does not mean there is no diagnosis. Primary menorrhagia and primary dysmenorrhoea are both diagnoses in themselves and there are options for support to manage the symptoms of both.
- Treatments available for primary causes include non-hormonal medications, hormonal-based treatments and non-medical approaches.

CHAPTER 4:

WHAT IS ENDOMETRIOSIS: THE SCIENCE

THE CHAMELEON OF GYNAE HEALTH

A chameleon is a creature known for its elusive nature – its ability to hide and go unnoticed and be hard to pinpoint and yet thrive unseen. There is a reason that gynaecologists have nicknamed endometriosis 'the chameleon of gynae health', because it too has an incredible ability to hide, be difficult to pinpoint and yet thrive as it causes havoc within a woman's pelvis and even beyond.

Knowing what I know now, I am amazed that in medical school this insidious disease was condensed into a simple description as being a 'disease which causes painful and heavy periods' – a gross disservice when considering the complexity of the organic processes at play or the life-changing impact it can cause for the woman affected. Suffice to say it is *not* just painful periods. It is an incurable disease process and for far too long women have not been given the explanation and tools they deserve to reclaim control of their health and life. Until now.

To understand how to navigate the lengthy process of receiving a diagnosis or the intricate options of how to manage this debilitating condition, we first need to understand what endometriosis is, why it happens and what it means to live with it. Before we dive into these elements in more detail, I want to share with you why it is important to have such a thorough, reliable explanation of what endometriosis is. Because I, as a doctor, failed to understand this disease for so many years and suffered the consequences, which is a huge reason why I am writing this book – so that you don't need to fall down the all-too-common pitfalls set up by this chameleon.

INTRODUCING ENDOMETRIOSIS

Endometriosis is gaining waves of coverage in the news, social media and online health forums, more than any other period-related disorder. Why is it that affected women have become so passionate about advocating to raise awareness of it and (metaphorically) scream from the rafters about its dangers? It might not be the most common of all the gynaecological diseases, but it has the biggest reputation.

The answer is because it is incurable and if it's mismanaged or diagnosed too late, it can cause life-long pain and disability as well as increasing the risk of miscarriage and profoundly impacting fertility and mental health.

While its recent coverage on social media will no doubt help to raise awareness, I fear that this deluge is drowning out the essential soundbites of reliable information and knowledge needed to more accurately support and empower women. Having the tools to make informed choices and regain control of our health and wellbeing is essential, yet for endometriosis this information is rarely visible, let alone viable.

To even begin to explain how to find support to manage such a complex disease, there are a lot of myths to debunk, and we need to go right back to the basics. I want to delve into endometriosis not just as a *disease process* within the pelvis, but also how this disease *affects the body*, the woman living with it and how treatment options have an influence on both the patient and the disease itself. I have therefore dedicated two chapters of this book to discussing the question 'What Is Endometriosis?' This chapter looks at what endo is as a disease, while Chapter 5 will look at what endo means for someone living with this incurable condition.

My story

I have advanced endometriosis as well as quite a few other health conditions. Within the world of endometriosis my personal 'situation' is thus: I am 37 and despite having had my uterus, ovaries, fallopian tubes and cervix removed, I still have ongoing active disease (i.e. there are still remnants of disease that are sticking my organs together, causing prolapses, adhesions and bowel and bladder damage). I need equipment to empty my bladder and my bowel. I've had six miscarriages, more than five surgeries (honestly, I've lost count), a round of IVF, a uterine fibroid (which was identified at some point and included in my notes, but no one told me and led to a major haemorrhage during an emergency caesarean), a premature traumatic birth and postnatal depression. I am in menopause and showing signs of early osteoporosis. My libido is far from what it used to be and my sleep patterns are extremely erratic, as is my memory and stamina.

I feel like I have a body of a 70-year-old woman some days. This is largely because of my endometriosis being mismanaged by my medical team early on, and partly because I was not equipped with the knowledge to advocate or make informed choices for myself.

I am the classic cliché of someone who had red flags from my very first period but who did not get a diagnosis for another 15 years. I was put on the pill like so many women for dysfunctional periods, without explanation, and encountered numerous instances of mismanagement and failings along the way. I have experienced what many women describe as 'medical gaslighting', medical misogyny, possibly even neglect at times.

I have experienced the social stigma of endometriosis; I have had to change my entire career, family choices, personal lifestyle and self-identity because of it. I am a very different person from who I thought I would become – a stronger version of myself I could never have before imagined. I have taken a career path that, although different, is one I love and find truly rewarding. It is for this reason that I continue to advocate for always finding hope and the importance of accessing tools to thrive, not just survive (with any diagnosis).

> **The wider impact**
>
> Endometriosis doesn't just affect the person going through it – their partner and family are also along for the ride. As hormonal treatments are changed frequently like a pick'n'mix cocktail, it can feel at times like medics are blindly throwing them your way until something sticks. It can also feel that there is little to no thought on the consequences for you as a person being influenced mentally by these hormones. How you are with the world around you – both in how you engage and how you are received while you are going through this – is also massively inhibited by society's lack of understanding.

I am not alone in my story or experiences. I know full well the extent to which this disease can exert disruption, pain and upset into one person's life. What I also know is that so much of my experiences could have been avoided if:

- The medical teams I encountered along the way had been fully equipped with the knowledge to diagnose and treat endometriosis.
- I'd felt empowered to advocate for myself.
- The world around me understood the condition.

I am finally in a place of contentment with my health. I have worked hard to move beyond the 'why me' resentment at my body or diseases and the disenfranchised grief.

My emotions are a reasonable response to the trauma I encountered, but it's important for us all to let go at some point, regain control over our lives and have the freedom to truly live. So, I don't often like to 'look back' or think how things would be had something been any different. However, I recognize that my life's experiences are not an isolated occurrence and that so many women have the same story. A story that does not need to be so long, full of unexpected turns and dramatic twist plots. This should not be a familiar story for so many women. This is not the story I want for my daughter or my friends, as it quite simply does not need to be anyone's story.

While the science and understanding is still young in understanding the full complexity if the disease, this should not be a barrier to being liberated from needless trauma and suffering.

While I now know that I was always destined to have a hysterectomy at some point, I also know that the number of miscarriages, the financial weight of having IVF that was destined to fail, the stigma and so much trauma I experienced could have been, without a doubt, avoided. I know that countless physicians made ill-informed (some may say 'wrong') decisions in managing my condition. I too made multiple wrong choices about my treatments and journey, all because I was not equipped with the information.

It has taken me over a decade to gather together all the answers and information about this disease. I can't change what has happened to me, but I wanted to really understand why there is still so much chaos and confusion, and why women are being let down repeatedly. I have looked and am truly appalled to see that there is no resource I can find *anywhere* that truly presents the full picture of this disease. Although advances are unfolding all the time, it's shocking to me that still no one has pulled together a comprehensive package of information to educate people – there is information out there, but it's scattered.

By sharing the full picture with you, I want to bring you *fully* into the world of endometriosis in all its complexity. Had I been presented with even a fraction of this information ten or twenty years ago, my own disease journey would have been vastly improved.

I have come to realize there are two different perspectives in understanding what endometriosis is, and both are equally important: what it is as a disease process and what it means to *live* with it. It is the gynaecological chicken and egg situation: they go hand in hand.

THE PHYSICAL DISEASE

> **Fast facts**
>
> Endometriosis:
>
> - Affects one in ten women.
> - Is a disease of painful periods (dysmenorrhoea) and infertility.
> - Can be associated with heavy bleeding.
> - Causes major disruption to quality of life.
> - Is incurable.

A simple but *inadequate* description is: endometriosis is an incurable gynaecological disease, causing pain and infertility. This is, in essence, the premise of teachings at medical school. Only doctors that go on to specialize in general practice or obstetrics and gynaecology will be taught more than this.

My knowledge of endometriosis was so limited in my medical training that not once did it occur to me that I might have it myself. I had normalized my own painful, dysfunctional periods for years, then had the symptoms masked by the contraceptive pill, so even as I was taking an exam on the topic, it didn't occur to me that I could be that patient.

A brief history

The first recognition of endometriosis dates to 1690, when early doctors and scientists first made descriptions of ulcers in the peritoneal cavity. In the 1700s it became recognized as a disease that causes pain, and then not much changed for about 300 years. The simplified view that endometriosis is simply 'painful periods due to ectopic lesions' has persevered far longer than needed, given the advancing technologies. Meanwhile, other conditions (some might say ones that are not solely female inflicting) have had a lot more funding, interest and enlightenment. While it is better late than never, we are now in a state of playing catch-up, which offers hope to future generations, even our current children, but offers little in way of compensation for previous generations.

Endometriosis does not play by the normal rules of pathology. It is a medical enigma that defies so many usual 'rules' of physiology, biology, anatomy and immunology. Add in the significant social stigma and the long-overdue validation of women's suffering for 300,000+ years, and you have a perfect storm for a triggering diagnosis.

Historically referred to as a term – a mere label – for painful periods, the name has become synonymous with this description. Yet endometriosis is incredibly challenging to diagnose, a disease process governed by hormones and compounded by a dysfunctional immune system – with the latter only just beginning to be scientifically understood. The way that endometriosis behaves can differ from woman to woman, with no predictability or easy way to measure it. Some women will have minimal physical disease with debilitating symptoms, others have advanced disease and no symptoms, and many fall somewhere in between. Hence the chameleon nickname; its behaviour, presentation and ability to elude capture (or diagnosis) make it somewhat of a medical enigma.

Endometriosis a relatively 'young' condition in our medical repertoire.

Why is endometriosis so misunderstood?

So many women are misinformed or confused about endometriosis, whether through misleading information online produced by well-intended advocates without medical experience, or a potential lack of adequate communication by the medical team.

The essence of what makes endometriosis tricky is not always clearly communicated to patients, and this lack of understanding has created a barrier between patients and doctors. In doing my own research to bridge the medical-me and the patient-me, I recognize that a significant factor causing confusion is that endometriosis is not a simple disease process. As a result, doctors without specialist training in the disease are not equipped with the tools to adequately communicate with their patients. This is not a failing, but something true of any complex specialist disease.

When I say that the disease process of endometriosis is more complex than other conditions, this is not to put endometriosis on a pedestal. It's more to try to lay a fundamental, foundational understanding to address the confusion in medicine, society and online. I hope by the end of this chapter it becomes apparent that a lot of the mismanagement (or what may appear as mismanagement) is because endometriosis is, comparatively speaking, so complex and scientifically unique. The medical support isn't there because the understanding and technology hasn't quite caught up with the true extent of what the disease is.

There are some health conditions that have a (scientifically speaking) beautiful complexity of anatomical abnormality or a clear physiological process that are almost enjoyable to learn about. Endometriosis is not one those. I often see gross simplifications online suggesting that endometriosis is the presence of rogue tissue in areas where it shouldn't be, which causes pain and infertility.

Why does endometriosis happen?

There are multiple theories as to *why* endometriosis occurs, but the exact science and knowledge isn't complete (yet). As for so many diseases, there are blended theories that it's partly genetic and partly random.

Genetics

Family history suggests that there is a genetic component. Women who have mothers and grandmothers with the disease have an increased likelihood of experiencing it themselves.

Retrograde menstruation

This occurs when the period travels back through the fallopian tubes and into the pelvis instead of being expelled through the cervix and vagina. The endometrial cells then attach to the tissue nearby and start the process of endometriosis.

Secondary health conditions

Women with hypermobility, neurodiversity and other period disorders seem to be at a higher risk of developing endometriosis, suggesting that there is an underlying connective tissue disease component. An increased understanding of this alongside further investigations of the autoimmune element to the disease will shed more light on the true nature of *why* endometriosis arises (which will, in turn, lead to better treatment options).

THE BASICS

Endometriosis occurs when endometrial-like tissue (such as the inner lining of the uterus) grows where it shouldn't. This ectopic growth outside of the uterus (around the uterus, gynaecological organs, ovaries, peritoneum and other organs) causes pain, scarring, adhesions and infertility. It is a disease that is very much a process influenced and determined by both the hormonal processes (endocrine system) and inflammatory processes.

If we revisit the anatomy discussed earlier, the uterus has three layers: the peritoneum (thin outer skin-like layer), the myometrium (muscular layer to help the uterus contract) and the endometrium (lining of the uterus). The endometrium itself has two layers: the base layer which stays constant and the active layer which thickens ready for implantation and sheds if no embryo is received.

Endometrial tissue is extremely hormone sensitive and grows rapidly due to its role in the menstrual cycle and reproductive process. It is one of the lead soloists of our reproductive orchestra and has its own distinct moment in the symphony – without it the whole process would cease to perform.

Endometriosis is the process where tissue that is very similar to the active lining of the endometrium grows elsewhere else in the body, usually in the pelvic region. This is where the description on page 78 comes from, although it fails to mention that these plaques growing outside of the uterus can be severely damaging.

I like to describe endometriosis as being like garden weeds. Weeds grow wild where you don't want them to and invade gardens. Endometriosis plaques are the weeds invading the beautifully kept garden of our peritoneal cavity. They respond to the hormonal changes of oestrogen and progesterone, they spread throughout the cavity if left unchecked and cause nearby organs to stick to them and to each other, forming adhesions and scarring. If they tangle around or inside the fallopian tubes, they cause blockages and interrupt the flow of eggs and sperm on their quest to find one another and produce an embryo. The very presence of these endometrial plaques triggers an immune response which can cause miscarriages.

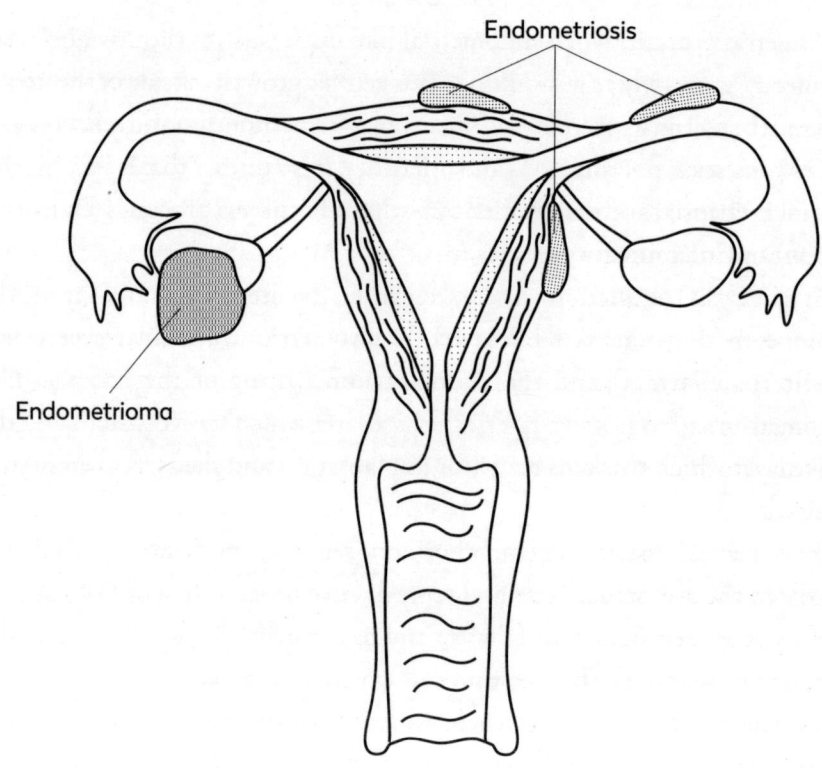

A unique and unpredictable disease

Endometriosis is caused by endometrial plaques – tissue that looks and behaves like that of the endometrium but growing outside of the uterus – but we need to understand *why* these tissues cause chaos for our bodies and minds.

Each women's experience of endometriosis will be different. Endometrial plaques could be placed into one hundred women and their experience and symptoms will vary as markedly as the personalities of the women themselves. Each woman's experience of having endometrial plaques will be different because this complex process of cell intrusion is influenced not only by hormones, but also by a woman's immune response. Some women won't develop endometriosis, others will but without symptoms and then there are those of us for whom the plaques grow rapidly and spread like wildfire. And even amongst the last group, some women might not have any discomfort, while others might be incapacitated with pain. Some might have miscarriages, some may not. There is no way of knowing how a woman will respond.

Endometriosis is a unique and unpredictable disease that is likely to be experienced differently from woman to woman, meaning there is no predictability in behaviour or outcome of how the disease will manifest or how to manage it. It has no obvious pattern and women with the same disease behaviour and symptoms could have very different responses to the same treatment.

This is often not properly explained when women are diagnosed. Endometriosis is simplified as a disease dominated by hormones, and as a result treatments tend to be hormone-targeted. But the reality is that this disease is a cacophony of hormones and immune system processes that interact differently for every single person.

Endometriosis is part endocrine disorder and part immune disorder. The body's immune system responds to different threats (such as infections, cancers and rogue cells) using different methods in the same way as a country might have air defences, sea defences and land defences.

For some women, a threat detected by their immune system can cause it to malfunction, and this is the case with endometriosis. The fact that endometriosis is also an immune disorder is often overlooked in resources and education, which has consequences for symptoms and treatment choices.

> An understanding that endometriosis is an oestrogen-dependent inflammatory disease rather than merely a hormone disorder is important for women and healthcare professionals alike when it comes to making decisions about treatment and the process of investigation, management and prognosis.

THE SCIENCE OF ENDOMETRIOSIS

There may be an instinct to skip the science bit and fast forward to treatment options. But given the complexity of this disease, an understanding of its anatomy is essential to make truly informed choices when it comes to treatment. If I had known the information presented here, it would have saved me a lot of pain, needless miscarriages and the heartbreak of IVF.

To feel empowered to advocate for our own health needs (which includes navigating the healthcare system) we need to be provided with as much information as possible.

I find that many health education materials online or within hospital settings are overly simplified. With some conditions this might be 'enough', but with complex conditions like endometriosis a lack of information opens the way for misunderstanding and can lead to women making decisions about their health without being in possession of all the facts. With this in mind, let's take a closer look at how endometriosis forms and behaves.

The endometrium

As we learned on page 25, within the inner layer of the uterus is the endometrium, which has a base layer that stays constant and a surface layer that changes in response to progesterone and oestrogen to become 'primed' for implantation. If no implantation occurs, it sheds away as a period comprised of blood, endometrial tissue and vaginal secretions.

This endometrial tissue is composed of ever-changing specialist hormone-sensitive cells which can encourage the growth of blood vessels and nerves as well as swelling and shedding depending on the environment (notably in response to hormones and inflammation as well as a host of other 'influential' messengers within the body).

Within the confines of the uterus, these specialist cells perform their duties and play a crucial role in menstrual and fertility health. But when they grow anywhere beyond the inner lining of the uterus, they are treated by the body as rogue intruders and treated in the same way as a virus.

Once the plaques begin to form outside of the uterus and the endometriosis disease begins, there is no cure and there is no going back. How many plaques form, their location and how they behave dictates the extent of the disease and disruption experienced by the woman. Like any avid gardener will know, you can use all the weedkiller in the world, but once those seeds find their way into foreign soil, it's a relentless battle of weed management. This is essentially the case with endometriosis.

The endometrial plaques

The plaques themselves can, scientifically, have lots of different appearances, names and descriptions. They can vary in size, depth and location, all of which influence how the disease behaves and the symptoms experienced. When undergoing investigations for endometriosis, your doctor will look at how wide the plaques are, their surface area and *depth*. Some rest lightly on the surface of organs or pelvis tissue, whereas some can invade much deeper, much like plants with superficial roots versus those with very deep roots. Where these plaques 'make their bed' can influence how the woman experiences the disease.

Where the plaques form

The are four main areas where the endometrial plaques form, and subsequently where endometriosis is then found:

1. Outside of, but on or close to the **peritoneum** of the uterus. These plaques commonly begin on the outside of the uterus (e.g. the fallopian tubes). When endometrial plaques/endometrial-like tissue forms inside the muscle layer of the uterus, the disease is known as adenomyosis (see page 201). *Adenomyosis is a separate diagnosis because the disease is situated in the muscle layer of the uterus, causing a very different clinical picture. Some women have endometriosis without adeno and vice versa; some women can have both.*
2. On and within the **ovaries**, where the plaques form cysts that fill with blood and endometrial-like tissue (endometriomas, also known as chocolate cysts). If untreated, these confined cysts can swell and enlarge, causing pain and infertility as well as increasing the lifetime risk of ovarian cancer.
3. **Deeper within the pelvis**, attached to the walls of the peritoneum and in gaps between the uterus and the bowel and bladder, where the disease can cause serious organ damage, resulting in blood visible in urine and stool (poo). For some women, the extent of the invasion into the bowel can be significant enough to need a bowel resection/stoma.
4. **Beyond the pelvis** to other organs is rare but can occur in places such as the lungs, diaphragm and (rarely) the brain. While not as common, this is the point where endometriosis becomes a full-body systemic disease with life-threatening complications.

My story

The extent of my own endometriosis is that of deep-infiltrating disease. The endo is attached to so many organs that my bladder periodically spasms and doesn't respond properly to brain signals, so I often must catheterize to empty my bladder.

> Years after having a hysterectomy, my bowel can still be extremely painful, and my multiple surgeries have left me with prolapses, distended bowel falling into places it shouldn't, making it difficult to empty without intervention or assistance.
>
> While not medically proven, I am certain that I have endometrial tissue in my nose as, when I was still menstruating, I would have cyclical nose bleeds. I always knew when my period was about to begin to the minute because I would have a problematic nosebleed every single month.
>
> When pregnant, I continued to bleed through my pregnancy. Far too many times I was told that endometriosis goes into remission during pregnancy and some surgeons refused to address the ongoing spotting and irritable uterus that was creating an increasingly problematic (and traumatic) pregnancy. I knew the spotting was endometriosis/oestrogen-related because whenever I had vaginal bleeding, my nose would also bleed. I refrained from pointing this out to my doctors for fear of sounding totally crazy at a time of immense stress, but it was evidence enough for me to know that the vaginal bleeding was indeed hormone related.

Is endometriosis cyclical?

Endometriosis is, without a doubt, a hormone-dependent disease. The endometrial plaques are extremely oestrogen and progesterone sensitive, and oestrogen fuels their growth. But an often-asked question is: are the plaques essentially bleeding internally and causing mini monthly periods within the pelvis? And therefore, are the symptoms of endometriosis women experience cyclical? Or more so – is it right that some clinicians may dismiss a woman's symptoms on the grounds of whether it is cyclical or not?

It is a very reasonable thought given the understanding that the plaques are formed of tissue that is similar to that of the uterus, which inevitably sheds each month to form the period.

The answer is that these endometrial plaques are formed of endometrial-*like* tissues. They can behave very similarly, and research has shown that for *some* women (or even some plaques within the same woman) the plaques *do* respond and behave cyclically, i.e. they have a pattern of swelling and bleeding each month. This blood then has nowhere to go because it is not inside the uterus with a designated exit point through the cervix and vagina. But the blood from the endometrial plaques is not a mini period because a period is more than just the shedding of these cells (see page 15). But the plaques can and do bleed within the peritoneum, causing a multitude of problems.

The blood they release accumulates, settles and causes an internal reaction by the body which accounts for so much of the pain. This blood also then helps seed and spread the endometriosis plaques further (like weeds in a garden). The blood is identified by the body as an intense irritant and it responds with inflammation, which in turn can cause adhesions and scarring.

So, for some women endometriosis will inevitably be cyclical, particularly for those in whom the endometrial plaques are bleeding each month in a cyclical manner. But the pain women experience isn't just caused by the blood itself. There are so many different aspects of this disease that cause pain, and many but not all will go into remission for two or three weeks a month. My pain and symptoms were initially cyclical, but as my disease progressed I found myself having pain every single day, sometimes worse than others, and there was no way I could have described it as cyclical. A misunderstanding of whether symptoms should or should not be cyclical is one of the main reasons endometriosis is so often misdiagnosed.

PHYSIOLOGY

I once heard a builder compare the human body to a house, and this analogy lends itself to understanding how the systems of our bodies work in tandem. We have the plumbing (the circulatory system) pumping blood through our vessels like the water and drainage system in the house.

The endocrine system manages our hormones, governing all areas of the body to keep the different systems running (sort of like Wi-Fi connecting all the rooms of the house). Then we have a central app (our brain) that connects all the different communication devices, receiving messages from the detection devices in our hormones and linking them to our defence system – the immune system.

The immune system responds to threats and has different tools in place to prevent an invasion from killing us, removing the threat from our bodies and repairing the damage caused. Every day our cells misbehave, and our body can even detect potential cancer cells and remove them without us ever knowing this has happened (cancer happens when our bodies fail to eradicate these cancer cells and they 'escape' our own defend-and-repair system: our immune system).

Endometriosis plaques are governed by our endocrine and immune systems, and the way these two systems interact creates a complicated process that is not easy to fix. Endometriosis isn't just the failing of one system; both the endocrine and immune systems have a role in this disease.

Research to date has largely focussed on the hormonal role of endometriosis, as the disease is fuelled and encouraged to grow by oestrogen. While a link to the immune system has been clear for a long time, we are only just beginning to fully understand its role. Research has now pivoted to explore in greater depth the full extent to which our immune system has a role in the process of endometriosis, which promises for more targeted treatments on the horizon.

The endocrine system

Endometriosis plaques are completely dependent on hormones, notably oestrogen. As the plaques are formed of cells similar to those found in the uterus endometrial lining that are designed to swell and grow in preparation for a potential embryo to implant, so the plaques also respond to oestrogen in the same way. As oestrogen circulates in our blood to stimulate the uterus lining, the plaques detect the rising oestrogen and grow and behave in a very similar way to endometrial cells. So essentially, oestrogen encourages the growth and spread of endometriosis.

But oestrogen doesn't simply encourage the plaques to become wider or deeper. Along with other hormones, oestrogen encourages new blood vessels to form (which then bleed, causing the disease to spread, resulting in more pain) as well as new nerve cells. These processes (angiogenesis and neurogenesis) are painful, while also adding to the physical damage and severity of the disease, making it harder to manage.

Another crucial detail about oestrogen is that while it fuels the plaques to grow, it is also a big factor in how we detect and experience pain. Oestrogen also increases the sensitivity of our pain receptors. So higher levels of oestrogen can make some women more sensitive to pain, triggering the smoke alarms of our metaphorical house. This is why many women find that having a tattoo, piercing or blood test while on their period can hurt more than at other times of the month.

This is a very significant missing piece of the puzzle that is not covered in educating people about endometriosis.

Oestrogen amplifies the pain signals, often disproportionately, to disease activity as well as fuelling the disease growth itself.

We have various pain receptors and pathways throughout our body. Together, they form a motorway-like network of communication to alert our brain (remembering we are primal evolutionary beings hard-wired for survival) to the presence of any potential threat. Survival mechanisms are in place to respond quicker than we can sometimes consciously react to protect us from harm. We need our pain receptors to alert us to any discord or threat to our bodies (inside and out).

Our experiences of pain are relative and vary from person to person. If our pain receptors fired off at a level ten regardless of the trigger, we wouldn't be able to cope and our reaction to minor aches and pains would be out of proportion to the threat. Worse still, if we had an under-reaction to pain (level one), we might not take our pain seriously (e.g. we might continue to walk on a broken leg). This type of pain response – i.e. the worse the pain, the worse the underlying problem – is what we, as humans, have come to know and understand. Makes sense, doesn't it?

With endometriosis, however, these rules of pain being proportionate to threat are completely and utterly ignored. The degree of pain being experienced is *not* proportionate to the disease severity because of the way that it's linked to oestrogen. The oestrogen doesn't just 'slightly increase the sensitivity of pain' – for some women it puts the body into level ten alarm that is irrefutably impossible to ignore. This could be in response to mild disease activity or significantly advanced disease activity – i.e. a level 10 warning regardless of actual threat.

Imagine our pain receptors are like smoke detectors, designed to sound the alarm in response to pain instead of smoke. Whereas most smoke detectors have one volume regardless of how much smoke is produced, imagine if their volume was proportionate to the size of the fire. A tiny match being lit wouldn't sound the alarm; burning toast would cause a quieter alarm; the kitchen being on fire would trigger a full-volume alarm; and the house being on fire would be loud enough to wake the whole street.

What oestrogen is doing in this context is creating a full-street alarm in response (sometimes) to what is the equivalent of a match being lit. Some women can have one small endometriotic plaque (minding its own business, not tangling organs, not affecting fertility necessarily) but the oestrogen causes an over-reaction of pain receptors. For some women a small plaque of this size would cause a small amount of discomfort, but for others their pain response is malfunctioning and causing an overwhelming, debilitating and unnecessarily disproportionate response.

It is for this reason that some women have endometriosis with no symptoms whatsoever. Their bodies do not have this hypersensitive response to the presence of oestrogen and so don't even register the presence of the endometriosis plaque. These women include those with a few, small plaques as well as those with widespread endometriosis.

For one woman the presence of a small plaque could be enough for her to be unable to work because the pain is all consuming and her brain is receiving a 'house on fire' alarm, while another woman who has endometriosis spread throughout the peritoneal region may present in the same way.

The pain is not proportionate to the disease activity.

You may need to re-read that sentence a few times to let it sink in. It took me a lot of reading and studying to get my head around this biological enigma of diseases. Our pain pathways – a survival instinct designed to keep us alive – are essentially gaslighting us. These pain pathways are telling us something is devastatingly wrong, causing our bodies to respond with the stress hormone cortisol, putting us into fight or flight mode. All over a metaphorical match being lit.

It is this process that causes some women to be cautious about taking pain relief to 'mask the pain'. As human beings we don't like to mask our symptoms and will often refuse painkillers until we know what is causing the pain. It may seem totally asinine to not want to mask pain, but this makes sense from a survival instinct; we want to remain in control because we don't want to switch the smoke alarms off. In most circumstances, we'd need to be alerted to pain getting worse because it would suggest the disease is getting worse.

I refused so many painkillers because of this misunderstanding. I didn't want to mask the pain because I wanted someone to find out what was going on. When the pain was getting worse, I genuinely thought this was a sign that my disease was getting worse. I felt emotional, frustrated and in disbelief that I was being offered more and more painkillers, and that I wasn't being taken seriously. It wasn't until years later that I came to understand that the severity of my pain was not an indication of disease severity, nor a reflection of imminent danger within my pelvis. It was due to the way oestrogen affected my experience of pain.

I see women complaining on social media that they are being fobbed off with pain relief rather than being taken seriously, all because they haven't been given this information.

The immune system

As if it wasn't enough that our endometrial plaques have gone rogue and the oestrogen circulating in our systems has heightened our sensitivity to pain, now our immune system, which is theoretically designed to detect inappropriate activity such as this, has somehow become very confused.

Our immune system is our body's defence and repair system (see page 92). In endometriosis, some of the processes designed to protect us, or the overall process of our immune system, becomes dysfunctional – to what degree varies from person to person. Some people have robust immune systems (those who rarely catch a cold), while others have immune systems that can't recognize an intruder from its own cells. These people usually have a medical history of autoimmune disease, and an allergy list as long as your arm.

With endometriosis, the body's immune system fails or becomes dysfunctional in varying ways; failing to recognize the disease, failing to stop it from spreading or failing to repair the damaged tissue. However, the immune system does recognize that *something* is going on and so sets off the red sirens and beacons for help, attracts all the different response teams to try to do *something* but as a result it creates more problems. The swarming of these different response mechanisms creates an inflammatory reaction which in turn causes more pain, more swelling, more scarring and more problems.

What's worse is that this immune process not only fails to fix the issue, but for some women this high state of inflammation in the pelvis causes issues throughout the body. The high inflammatory state can trigger the onset of other disease processes or exacerbate existing one. This is why some women describe symptoms that may be dismissed by doctors who don't have a specialist interest in endometriosis, such as joint pain, muscle aches, fatigue and headaches. While these symptoms might not have an obvious link to endometriosis, the inflammatory process happening throughout the body means the impact extends beyond the pelvis.

As a result, women who already have other autoimmune diseases may notice that the symptoms and disease activity of their other conditions will be considerably worse during an endo flare, or if the endometriosis disease is not adequately managed. The worse the endometriosis/inflammatory response to the disease, the worse the other autoimmune disease may become.

What's more, if someone is prone to having a dysfunctional immune system, the presence of endometriosis might be enough to push someone's immune system over the edge and increases the risk of developing other autoimmune conditions, such as:

- Lupus/systemic lupus erythematosus (SLE)
- Sjögren's disease
- Raynaud's disease

- Rheumatoid arthritis
- Autoimmune thyroid diseases (over- or under-active)
- Multiple sclerosis
- Inflammatory bowel disease
- Addison's disease

At present, endometriosis is not officially classed as an autoimmune disease because there is no obvious, distinct pathway of dysregulation, but the science is catching up.

When researching material for this book, I had a real eureka moment. I was diagnosed with endometriosis around the same time as I was diagnosed with lupus. I was experiencing secondary infertility and so went down the pathway of being tested for everything. I'd had multiple miscarriages and had painful joints, rashes, as well as horrendous period pain. I was sent down two very different pathways:

- A gynaecology referral, which lead to an endometriosis diagnosis and treatment.
- A rheumatology referral, which lead to a lupus diagnosis and treatment.

The two specialities weren't particularly interested in the coincidence that both conditions had suddenly become problematic at the same time in my life.

There is a rule in medicine – Occam's razor – which states that the simplest explanation is usually the answer. It is explained to medics that the chances of an individual having two very different unrelated diseases spontaneously present at the same time is very unlikely. Yet there I was for nearly a decade being treated for these two separate conditions, having absolutely no clue that they were related. Endometriosis probably exacerbated or set off the other new autoimmune conditions I was then diagnosed with.

I now look back and realize my lupus symptoms (which had been present since I was about 18, incidentally the time my periods became more problematic) had become worse as my endometriosis got worse. Both medical teams began their individual approaches – I had multiple surgeries for the endometriosis and was started on immune-regulating medications for lupus. I felt well, I fell pregnant – which treatment therapy was the solution? Both.

I admittedly got very over-excited upon discovering this and, knowing my own body and personal journey with my autoimmune medications, I know the specific cells in my immune system which misbehave (based on which therapies have helped improve my joint systems). I then investigated where research on endometriosis is now headed and, sure enough, the connection between these specific immune processes and endometriosis is now being explored further. The medication treatments I was on that helped my autoimmune disease potentially also helped my endometriosis.

This is hugely exciting as it shows promise for the future of women living with endometriosis. Until the last few years, all funding and research has been entirely focused on hormones and blocking the oestrogen pathways linked with endometriosis. Now, finally, the research is turning to altering our immune systems to stop the inflammatory processes to try to downgrade the war to a minor conflict – or even, one dare hope, a ceasefire or peace treaty.

The link between hormones and the immune system

It is this link between our hormones and our immune system that explains why endometriosis behaves differently from most other diseases, with no consistency from woman to woman. It also explains why the treatment pathways aren't straightforward – because how each woman's body responds to their disease is entirely different from one to the next.

Returning to the orchestra analogy, in our bodies we have the conductors – oestrogen and progesterone – telling the musicians what to do. Imagine there are some rogue musicians in the audience who brought their own instruments along. These are the endometrial plaques – rogue tissue appearing where it's not meant to be and responding to the hormones by growing and causing more problems.

Some online resources will leave the explanation there, but the immune system also plays a significant role in the process. We have rogue musicians uninvited and misbehaving, so the security guards – our immune systems – step in, *but* rather than approach the musicians directly and try to remove them (as would normally be the case), the presence of the intruders – the endometrial plaques – is so sneaky that they cause chaos amongst the security. Instead of responding to the inflammatory response, the immune system ends up causing more adhesions, making the situation worse.

And the disruption doesn't end there. The third layer of this escalating gynaecological crisis is that for some women (not everyone, because remember there is little consistency with this disease) oestrogen has a delightful side-talent for increasing the sensitivity of our pain receptors (see page 90). So, while oestrogen is conducting the reproductive system, for women with endometrial plaques the oestrogen is also fuelling the growth of these lesions. For some women (often those prone to a dysfunctional immune system) the presence of these plaques causes an inflammatory response, making the situation worse. Then for more women still – there is an added layer of chaos when the oestrogen not only spurs on the endometriosis, but the oestrogen itself causes a disproportionate pain response.

Layer after layer after layer of chaos. Imagine a cartoon scenario of an incompetent conductor trying to get music from a band with broken instruments. Then the audience begin chiming in. Incompetent security guards come in blindfolded, unsure who to attack and how. Then to complete this chaotic scene, the conductors set the smoke alarms off. This would be funny if it wasn't the reality of what is happening inside the precious, sensitive reproductive territory of women's bodies.

STAGING: DOES SIZE MATTER?

Staging is something that is important with any disease, more so for the medical teams. It is a way of grading how severe the disease is in physical presence and how much damage and disruption it's causing within the body. Staging is commonly recognized for grading cancer, particularly for differentiating between curable and incurable (or metastatic) disease. Even types of bone fractures have a staging system.

Staging is a way of quickly communicating between doctors a disease activity in terms of physical damage/spread. The staging process for endometriosis is similar but can be a cause of confusion for some patients and I will shortly explain why.

My story

By the time I was undergoing surgical procedures for endometriosis, I'd been experiencing the worsening of pain every month for about two years. I couldn't understand why every month I felt like I was being slowly killed from the inside, and no one was listening. The rising panic that something must be catastrophically wrong was exasperated by the seeming lack of urgency from my medical team. At that point I was totally ignorant of the oestrogen pain hyperreaction (see page 90) that can be a feature of endometriosis. When I woke up from my latest surgery, the consultant came to tell me he had found multiple endometrial plaques and what he had done with them.

The first words out of my mouth were: 'Is it stage four?' My consultant rolled his eyes and smirked, 'Yes, Liz, it is.' I felt so vindicated that the stage of disease, in my ignorant mind, reflected the pain I was experiencing. I honestly thought I was losing my mind because the pain was so suffocating, and I was terrified of waking up to be told there was very little disease evident. Because after years of already feeling like there was something wrong with me for not being able to cope with periods that society was telling me were 'normal', I didn't now want to be told that yes, I have this disease, but it's 'not that bad' and my pain perception was an over-reaction.

But that was me being completely ignorant of the truth. I could have very easily been one of the women waking up to be told they have stage one endometriosis.

Some women might feel fortunate to be told their disease is in stage one, but they might not be told that the stage of disease has no bearing on the reality of the pain they are experiencing. They almost certainly won't have been told about the oestrogen pain hyperreaction (see page 90). We are still in a situation where there is inadequate training and understanding of endometriosis, even amongst gynaecologists (let alone GPs). This means so many women are still left feeling utterly alone, humiliated and bereft as to why they have what is deemed as a stage one disease, but they are unable to work because of pain. If the medics and patients are confused, imagine trying to explain this to an employer.

Fast forward several years and while researching endometriosis in more depth, I became really confused by what appeared to be a major scientific error. Research paper after research paper discussed the development of yet another new hormone-based drug, but all that was being described was how effective the drug was in reducing a patient's experience of pain. None of these drugs was seemingly targeted at reducing the growth or size of endometrial plaques, and I couldn't understand why. Then it dawned on me: size does not matter. Most of the current non-surgical treatments available were not trying to directly shrink the lesions, they were trying to improve the quality of life by reducing the pain symptoms associated with the disease.

The reason for this is twofold:

1. The size of the plaques, and therefore the staging of the disease, is not proportionate to symptoms, so research effort goes into what is ultimately more important to women: their quality of life.
2. At present, endometriosis cannot be cured, so most treatments are aimed at mitigating the damage caused (which, in the absence of a cure, is the next best thing).

The use of language around staging and the confusion about how staging affects pain (or not) can be upsetting for many women. Staging does, however, provide important recognition of how advanced the disease is in terms of organ damage and long-term complications, so it is useful for monitoring disease progression. But in terms of acknowledging the full picture and impact of endometriosis on someone's life, the current staging system is inadequate.

> **Stages of endometriosis**
>
> A commonly used staging system for endometriosis is the ASRM (American Society for Reproductive Medicine) system. It's important to remember that staging categorizes how much disease is physically present and where it is – it's not a reflection on symptoms and the impact on the woman as a patient.
>
> **Stage one – minimal**: Few small plaques close to or around the uterus.
> **Stage two – mild**: More evidence of disease in number and/or size of plaques further away from the uterus and onto distant peritoneal tissue.
> **Stage three – moderate**: Multiple, larger plaques further spaced and growing deeper into the underlying tissue. Possible presence of ovarian cysts (endometriomas) with extensive adhesions.
> **Stage four – severe**: Deep infiltrating disease, large ovarian endometriomas, extensive adhesions and other organ involvement.

CHAPTER SUMMARY

You may by now appreciate just how complex endometriosis is. I truly feel that a diagnosis of this incurable disease should be accompanied by counselling and a reasonably thorough explanation.

So many of the hidden truths of the disease – the fact that the pain is disproportionate to the disease size, or that the inflammation causes other symptoms – mean women are not able to understand the treatment options available to them and aren't having adequate conversations with their medical team.

Key takeaways

- Endometriosis is a complex disease characterized by endometrial-like tissue (uterine lining tissue) growing outside of the uterus, causing inflammation, scarring and adhesions.
- The disease process is fuelled by hormones (namely oestrogen) and exacerbated by a dysfunctional immune response.
- Endometriosis is incurable and symptoms include severe pain, organ damage and infertility.
- There is currently no way to predict how any woman's individual disease activity will behave, how fast it will progress and how severe it will become.
- Staging is useful for medical and surgical teams to grade the physical spread of disease and organ involvement, but it can be entirely disproportionate to the degree of pain a woman experiences and the impact on quality of life.

CHAPTER 5:
LIVING WITH ENDOMETRIOSIS

SYMPTOMS AND SIGNS

When we describe a disease in terms of the process – the anatomical changes, the clinical pathology – we ignore the important aspect of what this means for the patient.

Endometriosis is often dismissed as a disease of painful periods, but this description is completely inadequate. This is a disease that is far more than 'just' pain. Some descriptions will also mention that endometriosis can cause infertility. Very true, but again this fails to communicate the full impact of what a diagnosis of endometriosis can potentially mean to a woman's day-to-day life.

After reading Chapter 4, you may have a renewed appreciation of just how much devastation endometriosis can cause and how little it's understood and managed by clinicians, let alone patients. This is beginning to improve and will continue to do so as research finally shifts towards the autoimmune aspects of the disease.

As with most conditions, a diagnosis is nothing without an explanation of what it means in terms of its impact on a person's life. Within medicine, as clinicians we are familiar with being taught what the signs and symptoms are for any disease.

- **Signs** are the physical manifestations of a disease – the visible changes on a body or to bodily functions.
- **Symptoms** are what the patient experiences (e.g. nausea, tiredness, pain).

Having been both doctor and patient, I have come to recognize that there is an aspect that goes slightly beyond the symptoms, and that is the *impact*. Patients not only need to know what symptoms they may face, how tired they might be and what level of pain is to be expected, but also whether fertility is going to be more difficult and how likely it is they can continue their job.

Some conditions, like cancer, come with a consultation of 'breaking bad news' – sitting the patient down and explaining not only what the cancer is but also what this means for the patient. What their world will look like in the immediate now and in the short- and long-term future. A life-changing condition has life-changing consequences, which need to be explained to a patient so that they are fully informed and can process what is happening within their body. However, this kind of explanation is often sadly missing for women when they are told that they have endometriosis.

Whether you are early on in your menstrual journey and need to know what to look out for, or years into your own battle of trying to get a diagnosis or understand how to manage your disease better, you need to know what the impact is for you as the patient.

Symptoms

- Pelvic pain
- Severe period pain
- Pain during or after sex
- Pain when passing poo
- Pain when urinating
- Difficulty conceiving
- Fatigue
- Bloating
- Low mood

> **Signs**
>
> - Blood in urine
> - Blood in stool
> - Bloating
> - Infertility
> - Miscarriage

When we consider the signs and symptoms, we need to keep in mind that endometriosis can sometimes be a cyclical experience or sometimes not (see page 87). Some endometrial plaques will respond in a cyclical manner, swelling and bleeding in response to the monthly surges of oestrogen, and so the corresponding pain will also be cyclical, but some plaques don't behave in this way and so symptoms can change on a day-to-day basis.

PAIN

Pain in the pelvis. Pain passing poo. Pain during or after sex. Pain pain pain. If you've ever had a migraine or horrendous toothache, you will know how it is almost impossible to work, concentrate or do anything else while experiencing that level of pain. It ruins your mood, your ability to find enjoyment in anything, and it's exhausting.

Not just period pain

What people often don't realize is that with endometriosis the pain isn't always just period pain. Endometriosis causes multiple different types of pain that all blur into one hazy cloud of suffering. First, there's the usual pain of the menstrual cycle, which is governed by prostaglandins and the pain associated with shedding the period. Secondly, there's the pain caused by the endometrial plaques essentially invading tissue, triggering the different types of nerve receptors. Thirdly, it's the bowel cramps and the inflammation causing a chemical 'sting' within the pelvis. Sometimes recognizing the different types and triggers (e.g. pain associated with pooing) can be useful in guiding a diagnosis, or even recognizing if the type of pain is changing over time.

We know that our bodies are programmed to pay attention to pain, and that the pain caused by endometriosis can be totally disproportionate to the size of the plaques and the severity of the disease (see page 90). Our cortisol levels rise and our whole body is permanently in a state of alert thinking something catastrophic is happening that we aren't responding to.

Something that is truly disappointing is the number of women who are prescribed antidepressants or labelled as having mental health problems due to showing signs of distress and/or an emotional response to chronic pain. There absolutely may be a low mood or symptoms of anxiety, but these are usually a result of the pain, which can be relentless. A woman is not necessarily experiencing pain because she has depression; she is more likely to be depressed because she is exhausted and overwhelmed by pain that is not being addressed or managed appropriately.

Pain during sex

If you manage to get a break from the pain (or life in general) and find yourself in a sexual encounter either with yourself or a partner, endometriosis doesn't give you a break here either. What might begin as a good day that is seemingly pain-free can lead you into trying to seize the opportunity and commence something that should be filled with pleasure. Intercourse, or the act of penetration, can physically put pressure on the scarring or adhesions and be extremely painful and set a flare off – robbing all enjoyment and totally killing the vibe. You might then avoid penetration, knowing that this will cause discomfort, and think this will avoid pain. If you are lucky enough to reach climax without pain destroying the moment, the act of having an orgasm (which causes small involuntary contractions within the uterus) can very quickly be followed by a wave of pain as the endometrial plaques are unsettled because of the orgasm-associated contractions. What starts as a wave of pleasure is immediately followed by a wave of pain. Talk about an anti-climax.

For some women, pain during sex might be the only time they experience pain. Some women simply adapt and avoid intercourse because it's too uncomfortable, with no awareness that this is because they have a disease.

Other causes of pain during sex

Pain during or after intercourse can be due to a multitude of reasons, including infections, pelvic inflammatory disease and even an incorrectly placed IUD (intrauterine device, commonly called the coil). New or longstanding pain during or after sex is a red flag, whether it's related to endometriosis or not. Make sure you are up to date with your smear tests and don't let embarrassment stop you from seeking medical help.

BOWEL

There are many women who were given a diagnosis of IBS (irritable bowel syndrome) who later discovered their symptoms were in fact due to underlying endometriosis. I suspect this is a very common occurrence.

IBS (irritable bowel syndrome): a misdiagnosis

IBS is a diagnosis that captures a syndrome whereby patients experience painful bowel cramps, bloating, excess gas and erratic bowel habits. Some people with IBS have episodes of constipation; others have diarrhoea or loose stools. There is no obvious underlying cause and it is usually meant to be a diagnosis of exclusion, in that the organic causes and other culprits have been investigated and ruled out.

Conditions such as inflammatory bowel disease (Crohn's or ulcerative colitis), in which there is a visible disease process happening that needs urgent treatment to manage and avoid damage, or cancer or coeliac disease need to be ruled out before a diagnosis of IBS can be made. These 'other' rule-out conditions have medication treatments and pathways that need to be explored.

IBS can be one of those heart-sink diagnoses for some when they feel like their very real, very problematic symptoms have been dismissed and given a label that feels like no label at all. IBS isn't a disease process that has an obvious mechanism, there's no test for it and no treatment. It is essentially a label for symptoms and a diagnosis of exclusion.

As a doctor, I have seen a number of women who have a diagnosis of IBS and then if probed it becomes clear they also have symptoms that suggest endometriosis. I feel so frustrated when this happens; because they don't have painful periods or an obvious endometriosis link, they have been told they have IBS and left to it with little support.

Endometriosis and the bowel

Endometriosis can affect the bowels. If the endometrial plaques, scarring or inflammation invade the bowel space (this is because the uterus and bowel are close neighbours within the pelvis) then bowel symptoms will occur. The bowel is a very sensitive organ and doesn't like being disrupted or having its space invaded. If inflammation is happening nearby, this can cause diarrhoea, bowel cramps or make it very uncomfortable or painful as it fills with poo, more so when trying to evacuate that poo. This then adds to the bloating and discomfort.

If endometrial plaques then attach to the bowel itself, this causes another layer of inflammation, and a different type of pain. Every time the bowel passes a poo it hurts, because its smooth membranes have painful lesions biting through the wall, causing inflammation and scarring. The bowel them spasms, bringing fluid and inflammation to protect itself, which can cause diarrhoea, horrendous cramps and bloating. This results in a list of symptoms which are quite often labelled as IBS, but IBS is meant to be a diagnosis that, medically speaking, means the symptoms have no other cause. For many women these bowel symptoms are a direct result of their endometriosis, possibly the only symptoms.

For some with very advanced disease, the endometrial plaques can even find their way through the full thickness of the bowel wall and cause bleeding within the bowel. This can be seen as blood mixed within the poo and can be cyclical (see page 87).

Involvement with the bowel is an advanced complication very much feared by endometriosis patients and recognized as a very serious advanced progression of the disease. Once the plaques break through or attach to the bowel this can cause life-threatening complications. For some women, the only option is to have part of the bowel removed, which can lead to the need for a stoma. This carries with it a level of disability, infection risk and lifelong disease burden that needs to be avoided with the correct management of endometriosis.

Avoiding bowel and bladder involvement and the need for a stoma is one of the main targets of endometriosis treatment (as well as managing pain and addressing any fertility challenges). The dysfunction and disruption to these organs can also be compounded by the surgical procedures themselves (see page 166). This is one of the reasons why women need to understand why the hormonal treatments and medication approaches are so important. While some women are quick to think surgery is the only option – and some people push anti-hormone myths and misleading ideas on social media – we need to recognize the value of utilizing all options available.

My story

I am testament to the fact that multiple surgeries can achieve great things, but had I known earlier that staying on the contraceptive pill could have slowed the spread of disease, I may not have the complications I do now. The cumulative scarring and disturbance caused by my multiple surgeries has affected the nerves to several organs. My hysterectomy created a massive empty space for the bowel and bladder to fall into, causing prolapses, twists and turns. As a result, my bladder and bowel don't function normally, not just because of the endometriosis but also because of the surgeries required to try to treat the endometriosis. Had I continued taking the contraceptive pill rather than stopping for many years, my endometriosis may not have spread quite as far and wide and I may not have ended up with such advanced disease.

BLOATING

A particularly cruel aspect of endometriosis is that while causing infertility, it can also make you so bloated that you look pregnant. And not just newly pregnant, but third trimester pregnant. There is nothing like a stab to the (metaphorical) gut to be asked 'how far along you are', when not only are you *not* pregnant, but the topic of your fertility is likely to be extremely triggering. This bloating is a result of the inflammation, bleeding, excess fluid and the bowels being antagonized.

My story

I will never forget an incident that happened to me while working in A&E. I had been on a two-year run of hormone treatments, steroids and multiple operations for my endometriosis and autoimmune issues. I had gone from a UK dress size 8 to a size 16, so I was already feeling rubbish about my body and my self-esteem was at rock bottom. I was swollen and looked about six or seven months pregnant, and I had not long returned to work after yet another miscarriage.

I was sitting by a patient's bedside taking her medical history. After finishing a pleasant conversation with her I stood up to explain the next steps of her care. Before I left the cubicle, she asked me, 'How far along are you then?', gesturing to my stomach. My heart sank because I didn't want to make her feel uncomfortable despite my own excruciating discomfort. Also, I didn't want anyone to overhear this mortifying conversation. Rather than say 'That's a really presumptuous, offensive, personal question to ask,' or better still 'I'm not pregnant, goodbye,' I stupidly made the situation much worse for myself to save my patient embarrassment and responded with 'Shhhh, not very far, no one knows.'

Why on earth I said this I do not know because her response was then (in an obnoxious shriek for the entire ward to hear): 'No one knows? Honey, what are you – pregnant with twins? How can no one know, look at the size of you!'

> Suffice to say I walked away and had a little cry in the toilet, but many years later I have learned to laugh about it. As many women with endometriosis will know, an endo belly looks very much the same as a pregnant belly.

MOOD

A woman's mood is a response to the ever-changing hormones, both naturally occurring and through the treatments being instigated, as well as a response to the chronic pain, anxiety, frustration, fear and fertility issues ongoing.

A woman's mood is not unstable or imbalanced and is instead responding to the very real and significant distress going on within her body. A woman's perception of pain is not exaggerated because she has anxiety or depression, and her mood will be impacted *because of* the disease going on within her body and the treatments being given.

Many of us with endometriosis have been faced with years of pain and crippling symptoms. We may have been trying to make sense of what the disease means for us while having our lives turned upside down because of the pain, fertility fears, frustration, an inability to have sex and the impact on our relationships. Then on top of that, we might have been trying various hormonal medications that make us even more anxious or tearful than usual. If this sounds like you, then of *course* your mood is going to be affected. You wouldn't be human if you didn't have an emotional response to this long-term low-level trauma.

Experiencing pain and chronic inflammation day in day out for days, weeks, months, even *years* is exhausting. The exhaustion and fatigue we experience with endometriosis are not solely because of the ongoing inflammation, but also from enduring pain for so long. This takes its toll. Imagine never having a pain-free day and then someone suggests that the pain is in your head because you are depressed. Unfortunately, this happens to far too many women. (See page 249 for how to support your mental wellbeing.)

INFERTILITY AND MISCARRIAGES

After pain, infertility is the second major impact associated with endometriosis. There are different ways in which endometriosis causes infertility, and you can turn to Chapter 8 to find out more about fertility and pregnancy.

Infertility, or struggling to conceive naturally, is both a sign and symptom of endometriosis. The data suggest that many women will conceive naturally, although it will likely take longer than expected (within two years is considered 'normal' for someone without disease).

The two types of infertility are primary and secondary (see page 173), but the ways in which endometriosis causes infertility are largely due to the anatomical changes. Adhesions, scarring and plaques can block or twist the fallopian tubes and obstruct eggs from being released from the ovary, or prevent them from travelling to the uterus to meet the sperm.

What's more, the physical presence of the plaques and the associated inflammation means the environment is particularly hostile and inhospitable. As we discovered on page 29, the endometrium is quite choosey about whether to receive a fertilized egg, not only due to the quality but also the state of the environment within the pelvis. Any hint of infection, anaemia or state of unwellness for the potential mother and it would be more of a risk to compromise the woman further by taking on board and committing to a nine-month pregnancy. In this case, the body will likely reject the fertilized egg.

SEX: DRIVE, DESIRE, JOY AND PAIN

Endometriosis is dependent on hormones, and as hormones are the influencers of our biological drive to reproduce, it is inevitably going to have an impact on sex.

Pain during sex (dyspareunia, to use the medical term) can refer to pain before, during or after intercourse (see page 104). But there is more disruption to a woman's sex life than just pain, and as this sensitive topic is rarely talked about, it can lead to even lower mood and isolation. But if a woman understands the full impact of this disease on all areas of her life, she can communicate this to her partner to minimize the possible impact upon their relationship.

So, we know that endometriosis can affect our sex lives, but what can be worse is that the hormone responsible for a peak in pain (oestrogen) is also a hormone responsible for increasing our libido – our sexual urges. While oestrogen is encouraging the release of an egg, it also makes us feel, look and act sexier in a biological drive to find a partner to potentially fertilize this chosen egg.

So, the cruel twist of fate here is that our hormones are willing and wanting us to have intercourse at a time when it is probably going to be the most painful. If you are also trying to conceive, there can be a real mix of emotions when the thing you're wanting and willing to do is met with your body making you suffer for it.

Sometimes the process of intercourse can be tolerated, or you find ways to enjoy sex without penetration. Bingo, you think you've found a loophole to avoid that trigger causing pain. But then even the joy of climax is taken away – what begins with waves of pleasure is immediately engulfed by a tsunami of pain. Those pelvic muscles and organs contracting with the orgasm are quickly whimpering under the plaques as the inflammation is disturbed. Nowhere, it may seem, is safe for a pain-free sex life.

But this isn't really an obvious and easy symptom to go to the GP with, is it? Unfortunately, not many doctors are forthcoming with asking about this, either.

Cue an increasing disinterest in sex, which can lead to an increasing distance between you and your partner, which can impact your mental health, self-confidence and ability to find joy in another area of life.

Medications

Taking painkillers might seem like a valid option, and perhaps you've been put on antidepressants to help with the mood response to this chronic debilitating condition. But both can and do influence libido and even our ability to orgasm. Women are often prescribed painkillers and antidepressants with no full disclosure that these drugs can, as a side effect, impact their sex drive and ability to reach climax. These are not reasons to avoid such medications entirely, but the decision to take them needs to be an informed choice based on what is more important to you.

Chemical or surgical menopause

If your disease has progressed to a point where you are put into a chemical or surgical menopause to manage your endometriosis, you can celebrate that the pain has reduced if not gone entirely, and the disease seems very well controlled. Brilliant. But now you might have little or no interest in sex because there isn't much of that sexy oestrogen coursing through your body. This doesn't happen for everyone I must add (and is certainly not to be used as a reason to exclude this as a management option – see page 231), but we cannot ignore the reality that hormones influence all aspects of us, including our libido, interest in and ability to enjoy sex.

When a woman is put into a menopausal state as a management option for endometriosis, often her libido takes a hit as a side effect. The body is not craving sex anymore and the desire and interest isn't always there. This can create issues for a relationship, particularly if communication isn't great. The warning that this *may* happen and safety netting the implications by counselling not just the woman but also her the partner can leave both feeling prepared and supported.

There is no easy solution here, but there are options, support and hope (see page 251). What is ultimately the most important aspect of the impact of endometriosis on sex is the need for effective communication. You should feel confident about discussing this with your medical team – they are trained to have these conversations. If you would rather change some of your treatment options, perhaps tolerating a little more pain to regain your libido, that is your choice and your medical team need to know. The ripple effect onto sex life, relationships and mental health can be made worse or safeguarded against by having an awareness of the reality and extent to which endometriosis can take its toll. Communication not just with your health care team, but also with your partner can be paramount to reducing the impact.

IMMUNE SYSTEM: A DOMINO EFFECT OF INFLAMMATORY TRIGGERS

As outlined in Chapter 4, the autoimmune aspect of endometriosis plays a very real, very important part. Beyond understanding the processes of an inflammatory reaction within the pelvis, it is important to know what this means in all areas of your body.

First scenario: you've never encountered an autoimmune condition or chronic inflammation before. You may be one of those people who remains relatively impervious to the immune knock-on effects of endometriosis. But for some individuals, endometriosis may be the first domino in a diagnosis-toppling effect of developing multiple autoimmune conditions.

As discussed on pages 92–96, the endometrial plaques trigger an immune response, putting the body into an inflammatory state. How marked this state is will vary from person to person, but the rise of the inflammatory cells (our defence and attack cells) isn't just detected within the pelvis, they are in our blood stream and 'knock on doors' in other parts of the body as they pass by. This is why some women notice joint pain, fatigue, lethargy and headaches.

A story I hear time and time again is that of women who start the process of being investigated for endometriosis and within a year or two find themselves also being diagnosed with multiple other autoimmune conditions.

Second scenario: any existing autoimmune conditions you have are made worse. If you were already aware of your 'other' autoimmune conditions, you may have noticed that one flare can trigger another. In times like this it really can feel like our bodies are working against us, and despite my protest that our bodies are hard wired *not* to kill us, with autoimmune conditions our bodies can behave a little rogue and do inadvertently work against us.

Thankfully, research is now beginning to finally explore the full extent of this connection. What we do know is that endometriosis can exacerbate existing autoimmune conditions as well as trigger the onset of new ones. The link is not fully proven as to *why* (scientifically speaking) this happens, but we do know that it happens.

> **The link to other autoimmune conditions**
>
> Women with endometriosis are more likely to be diagnosed with other autoimmune conditions, such as:
>
> - Rheumatoid arthritis
> - Sjögren's disease
> - Antiphospholipid syndrome
> - Autoimmune thyroid disease
> - Multiple sclerosis
> - Raynaud's disease
> - Lupus
>
> If one of those conditions isn't managed correctly (or overlooked and missed) then it can affect the others.

When I look back at those early days of getting diagnosis after diagnosis, I can see that when I had one of my autoimmune conditions better controlled, all of them seemed to improve. My conditions were treated in isolation (which is probably the case for many women) because this link is still not fully understood. But having spoken to those directly involved in the research, I can see that in the future the immune-related medical teams will work closely with the gynaecology team and our bodies' state of inflammatory chaos will be treated as one, leading to a faster arrival at better health and disease management.

HORMONE TREATMENTS

Hormones are underappreciated influencers whose reach extends beyond the ovaries and endometriosis plaques. Advances in research and understanding mean that we now recognize just how influential our hormones are. These chemicals circulate in our blood not only having a big influence on our ovaries and pelvic organs, but also on the receptors throughout the body which also respond to them. Consequently, when we alter the balance of hormones (by introducing hormonal treatments such as the contraceptive pill), we are affecting not just the endometriosis but also our metabolism, mood, desire, drive, weight, focus.

Remember that oestrogen is the sex-focused hormone that influences our energy, motivation and behaviours to encourage us to mate, while progesterone is the lazy, nesting and calming hormone. High oestrogen can also cause some people to be more irritable, perhaps a little too assertive, while conversely progesterone can induce anxiety in others.

It is no surprise, then, that a disease dominated by hormones that is managed by altering the natural balance of these hormones is also going to impact other areas of our life.

Mood

My story

After the pain and infertility, the biggest issue I faced during my time with active endometriosis disease was the mood disturbances. Having never had any major issues with mood before, I was plunged into five years of having my hormones changed every six months. Different types of contraceptive pill, chemical menopause, pregnancy, miscarriage, IVF, surgical menopause . . . I had no consistency of oestrogen, progesterone or BhCG (beta human chorionic gonadotrophin) from one week to the next and they certainly didn't mirror a state that the body comes to expect. Add in that I am particularly sensitive to progesterone and it became a very emotionally turbulent time.

This essentially subjected my body to extreme levels of high or low oestrogen, high or low progesterone, no hormones and pregnancy hormones. I didn't know whether I wanted to cry, scream, have sex or never have sex again, or I just felt anxious or depressed. My mood was not consistent and I had short bursts of energy, drive, motivation and confidence (the good old oestrogen coursing

> through my blood). I took on new career projects and ambitions that later, when the oestrogen was ripped away as I was pumped with progesterone, I not only didn't have the motivation for but became horrendously anxious about.
>
> With these hormones being switched like the flipping of an hourglass, I lost all control over who I was and where my emotions were. And what's worse, I had no idea this was all because of the hormone treatments.

What happened to me happens to so many women: we aren't given the correct information and are left to deal with the wide-ranging side effects of hormonal treatments without guidance. When women aren't equipped with the understanding that these changes will be happening, they can't communicate this with their partners, friends and family.

Keeping a mood or symptom diary is probably the most beneficial thing you can do. Tracking your mood, energy levels, attitudes and behaviours along with what hormones you are on can help you spot how you respond to them. This can help guide you to make truly informed choices about your hormone treatments later down the line. Even without being on hormone treatments, knowing your baseline emotional sensitivities in correlation with your natural menstrual cycle (oestrogen or progesterone spikes) can help predict how you will likely react to different hormone treatments.

I eventually recognized, the hard way, that progesterone on its own was a big no-go for my mood. Without the balance of oestrogen to neutralize the anxiety-inducing progesterone, I end up an anxious mess, a version of myself I had never experienced before. Had I known to look out for this early on in my disease journey, I could have avoided a lot of distress. Endometriosis is hard enough without hormones wreaking havoc on our mental wellbeing.

For those who are already more susceptible to PMS or PMDD (see page 56), or those who are neurodiverse (see page 117), the impact of hormone treatments on mood is compounded. I don't share this as a deterrent to hormone treatments (and will explain more in Chapter 6), but because having a clearer understanding of what to expect allows for preparation, support and understanding.

Weight

Hormones can play havoc with your metabolism. Oestrogen loves curves, because evolutionarily speaking this makes us more attractive to the opposite sex (thus increasing the chances of procreation) and puts us in a healthy body state for carrying a pregnancy. Progesterone loves us to be relaxed, comfort eating to store up reserves for pregnancy and not behaving recklessly or in any way that could jeopardize a pregnancy.

It is inevitable, then, that the hormone treatments used to manage the disease come with the risk (and very common) side effect of gaining weight. You're already bloated from the physical disease itself, you're feeling out of control and disconnected to your body, sex is less pleasant and now you're gaining weight. Weight then makes the joint pains worse and affects our mood and ability to exercise. If you're being pumped with progesterone your interest, motivation and energy to exercise is further inhibited. It's a vicious cycle.

ENDOMETRIOSIS AND NEURODIVERSITY

As a society, we are getting better at recognizing the extent of neurodiversity. Everyone's personality, way of thinking, approach to learning and experiencing the world around them is as unique as their DNA. For those who are neurodiverse, for example, ADHD (attention deficit hyperactivity disorder) or ASD (autism spectrum disorder), life is already difficult as our social structure is catered to a neurotypical way of experiencing life.

For those who are neurodiverse, the impact of these hormone shifts and the experience of pain and changes beyond our control can be even more overwhelming. Then trying to navigate the healthcare system, confusion of a disease which doesn't make sense and the widespread impact which hasn't been adequately communicated – this can all be even more isolating and lead to an even greater impact of disability.

Medical research is just beginning to unearth an overlap between neurodiversity, hypermobility and period disorders. While the cause is not entirely clear, a link between connective tissue changes in some women is suspected. As a result, we are discovering that neurodiverse women are more likely to have hypermobility, and women with hypermobility more likely to experience menstrual health problems such as endometriosis and PMDD (see page 58). Researchers are looking into the genetic causes and potential autoimmune composition of these conditions, while also helping to assess whether someone is more likely to have a diagnosis if they are already sitting within one or more of these three groups. It's still very early days but definitely something to be aware of and I'm watching with eager anticipation to see how this will influence the future management of these conditions.

Our medical services, understanding and support are poorly equipped for the neurotypical among us and haven't even begun to adapt to support the neurodiverse community. I wish I could offer a solution here, but I hope that awareness and understanding will help to remove the self-blame, relieve some isolation and lead to a better understanding, support and communication with those around us. If you have a suspicion of being neurodiverse or a confirmed diagnosis, you may begin to realize that some elements of the disease's impact are particularly overwhelming. Finding communities of others who can relate is always helpful for emotional support, and communicating your individual needs with your medical team is paramount.

QUALITY OF LIFE

The endometriosis journey is not just a physical one. Endometriosis is commonly considered to be a gynaecological or pelvic disease, and reference to it as a full body disease is often reserved for those who have endometrial plaques outside of the pelvis (in the lungs, for example). I disagree with this. The impact of the disease, hormones and inflammation mean this very much is a full body disease for everyone.

Material impact

The NICE guidelines for endometriosis clearly state that endometriosis can impact 'material quality of life' (it's worth noting that the NICE guidelines don't say this for every disease). This is because endometriosis, for the reasons outlined in this chapter, inevitably affect a woman's ability to work and thus inhibit her income.

When women are busy occupied with surgical procedures, appointments and trying to just *live (or survive)*, the notion of dating, marrying, studying or trying to ascend the career ladder are no longer a priority, or (for some) even viable. This is compounded by endometriosis not being fully understood by society, and employers not recognizing it as a disease which is a lot more than 'just painful periods'.

With the right understanding and support, women shouldn't need to be so negatively impacted, but as a society we are just not there yet. Imagine if employers had read this book. Perhaps they wouldn't challenge why a woman has asked to work from home for a few days while she finds a way to cope with the impact endometriosis is having on her life.

Disability

As with most disabilities, it's not the condition itself which is disabling but society's inability and refusal to adapt. A person who cannot get to the upper level of a shop is not disabled by their reliance on a wheelchair; they are disabled because the shop does not have a lift.

No one is disadvantaged by the world being more adaptable and inclusive. Parents pushing pushchairs are not considered disabled but greatly benefit from the presence of lifts or ramps. An employer who takes the time to allow for flexibility, empathy and understanding for an employee facing challenging health conditions only stands to *gain* by better employee results, commitment and longer-term engagement.

Endometriosis is not in itself (yet) a recognized disability under the UK's Equality Act 2020. However, if someone shares and explains how they are impacted and affected, it can be acknowledged and occasionally approved as a qualifying disability. This stands for both disability benefits as well as any occupational health discussions.

CHAPTER SUMMARY

Endometriosis is an organic disease-causing physical chaos within the pelvis through a complex process that has no consistent behaviour from woman to woman. This erratic disease behaviour goes some way to explaining why its presentation from woman to woman is variable, making it hard to diagnose and even harder to manage.

The reality of this being a disease influenced by both hormones and immune dysfunction means the approaches for treatment are varied, but knowing what is happening within our bodies provides the strong fundamentals needed for you to make informed choices about your care. While incurable, this does not mean you are without options for managing the disease. More importantly, these management options can begin at the onset of symptoms and overlap with any other potential underlying cause. Trusting the process and beginning treatments can be crucial to long-term protection from disease progression.

Key takeaways

- Symptoms are not proportionate to underlying disease activity due to complex physiological reasons. This means that endometriosis can present with debilitating symptoms despite having caused few physical changes, and conversely widespread physical disease with few symptoms.
- The impact of endometriosis is more than just pain or infertility. The state of inflammation and the fact that so many treatments are hormone based mean that this is very much a full-body disease and is not to be underestimated.
- Understanding what is happening with endometriosis, particularly that the pain is often a body's overreaction to a simple trigger (i.e. oestrogen causing a heightened sensitivity in our pain receptors) means that exploring all options for treatments is crucial to improving quality of life.

CHAPTER 6:
GETTING DIAGNOSED WITH ENDOMETRIOSIS

THE ROAD TO DIAGNOSIS

It's no surprise that a disease nicknamed 'the chameleon of gynae health' has become infamous for its long average time to diagnosis – at present it takes seven to eight years (possibly as long as ten years) for a woman to be diagnosed. This statistic is both controversial and misleading for many reasons: it is unclear whether this statistic is capturing the moment a woman first reports painful periods to then receiving her diagnosis of endometriosis, or from the point at which endometriosis is first considered officially by the GP. Another reason this statistic is misleading is that women are rarely referred for a diagnosis without being started on treatment. During those years there is a medically guided process of exploring treatments, using different investigations to explore other potential causes, many of which are more common than endometriosis. Thus, women are rarely left ignored for ten years without support, despite what the headlines may suggest.

One issue that may lengthen the route to diagnosis is that endometriosis symptoms overlap with many other conditions (see page 47). With nine out of ten women experiencing period pain at some point and only one out of ten having endometriosis, it is entirely reasonable that the first presentations of dysmenorrhoea (painful periods) are initially treated with medications rather than an immediate gynae referral. Even once a referral is made, endometriosis is not easily diagnosed and usually requires a surgical laparoscopy (in which, like any surgical procedure, there is an element of risk involved), therefore caution is utilized in this approach. The lengthy time for a diagnosis is not always a failing;

for the large part it is a risk-based approach guided by response to treatment. The important thing for you to realize is that you have a say in this process; if treatments aren't working, go back to your doctor. These conversations are just that: two-way conversations with you exerting your right as a patient to make informed choices.

My story

Looking at when I first presented to my GP with painful periods to receiving a diagnosis of endometriosis, it took me approximately 15 years. For 12 of those years I was, absolutely, being treated for 'painful and heavy periods' with the word 'endometriosis' *never* being uttered in my direction. When I finally began asking the question of potential endometriosis, I was told that I *couldn't have endometriosis because my symptoms were cyclical*, then a year later I was told that my symptoms *weren't cyclical enough*. I was told that family history is of no relevance, despite nearly every female in my maternal bloodline having had a hysterectomy in their early thirties for what was clearly endometriosis.

There are, without a doubt, lot of failings in the system contributing to poor management of women with confirmed or suspected endometriosis. That said we, as patients, need to trust our healthcare providers and, in turn, feel supported. The investigation process for endometriosis is a long and complex one and it can take an inordinate amount of time to go from 'possible endometriosis' to 'suspected endometriosis' before finally reaching 'confirmed endometriosis'. But with the right tools and knowledge you can and will navigate the process.

MEDICAL PATHWAYS EXPLAINED

Medical guidelines dictate that the journey of diagnosis runs right alongside starting treatment. You should not be wandering towards getting a diagnosis without being started on the various types of medications to help manage symptoms and disease activity, and here lies your first reason to slow down.

The way the NHS system is structured is that your day-to-day care is overseen by the GP, your community general practice. This first level of care is called primary care. The primary care setting is the go-to provider for general medical care and support. The GP/primary care setting can treat, arrange certain scans and investigations of which the *GP* arranges, looks at the results and can respond accordingly.

Being referred to a hospital specialist means being referred to secondary care – the next level/tier where the doctors are specialists in specific areas of medicine and see the more complex patients that need specialist input. Sometimes these specialists in secondary care will start medications/treatments and guide the GP how to manage this day to day and then check in once or twice a year. Sometimes these specialists in secondary care need to perform surgery or have a regular, closer relationship with the patient because their needs are more advanced/niche.

Then there is another level: tertiary centres. These centres are very similar (and probably experienced as the same to many patients) as secondary care. The difference being is that these house specialists within a speciality. Some tertiary centres are known for their advanced cardiac services, others for their neurology services. While most secondary care hospitals have consultants within the main specialities, there is a limit to the level of specialist treatments even they can provide.

Just like all doctors when leaving medical school have a little knowledge in most conditions, GPs go on to have a deeper knowledge of all conditions. Hospital specialists will train in one area. Obstetrics and gynaecology consultants will train in female reproductive organs and pregnancy (obstetrics being the pregnancy side, gynaecology being the reproductive organs when not pregnant). All gynaecologists are surgeons and will have some degree of training in endometriosis. However, while they could all technically do a laparoscopy to look for endometriosis, not all will have the advanced specialist skillset to be considered an endometriosis specialist.

The next important thing to highlight is that everything I write about in the next few chapters with regards to 'good medical practice' and 'what should be done' is based on the leading clinical guidelines which all doctors are strongly encouraged to follow, whatever the speciality. In the UK we have the NICE guidelines – a clinical library of 'how best to diagnosis and manage' nearly all conditions within health. These guidelines are regularly updated and written based on all the latest research going on in the world. For the most part, these are the framework for how doctors practise, either adhering very close to if not *to* these guidelines.

I also want to add that these processes have been written with the NHS structure in mind, and a lot of this structure is guided by the NICE guidelines and conducted in a way that is to optimize patient need with some consideration of resource availability. The processes may be different within a private route of care and vary between private practices – private practice is not regulated in the same way as the NHS.

First symptoms versus first suspicion

Asking a woman on the 'endometriosis pathway' when she first heard the word 'endometriosis' is different from asking when her symptoms first began. Both are equally important because, for many women, the time from those first symptoms and recognizing the potential underlying disease is not short.

I sometimes imagine endometriosis as a little weed-like gremlin in my pelvis, sitting back slightly smug. It creeps up slowly, building its web for the most part unnoticed because society is telling women that heavy and painful periods are 'normal'. Then when the woman finally is alerted to the potential presence, the media is telling her to be outraged that she isn't receiving an immediate diagnosis. But, as we now know, this disease doesn't behave in a way that makes it easily detectable and a number of other possibilities and diagnoses also need to be considered.

Endometriosis cannot be instantly diagnosed, and it does not *need* a diagnosis within two weeks. We have come to expect an urgency within the healthcare system that is not as relevant to endometriosis as many people would like or even have come to expect.

There are different ways in which you might come to the place of wanting or needing a diagnosis:

- You may be in the very rare category of being fairly young (under 20) and you've spotted the symptoms very early on in your menstrual life.
- You may be in your twenties, thirties or forties and have tolerated or even normalized relentless and debilitating periods for years. You have suffered in silence, you've screamed and cursed, you have a longstanding loathing and apprehension of the impending 'time of the month'. You may have even been trying to get pregnant, struggled to conceive or struggled with miscarriages. Either the GP has uttered the words 'endometriosis' to you somewhere in your many visits to them for your heavy and/or painful periods (my suspicion is not on the first ever encounter) or you've had a friend or seen a post (or read this book) and suddenly the lightbulb has gone on when you have read about endometriosis and realized you have the symptoms – and now what next?
- Or you may be the poor soul who hears the words 'endometriosis' for the first time after a scan or surgical procedure. You've gone through much of the investigation process totally unaware of the term and suddenly it's been landed on your doorstep. If this is you, I am sincerely sorry that the forewarning and counselling was not there to help you prepare. Read on for some reassurance about the journey you went through to get where you are.

Reassuring flags

The following pages deal with the process of investigating the underlying causes of symptoms to either rule in or out endometriosis. Here I point out what I call 'reassuring flags'. These are the opposite of a red flag and will hopefully relieve some anxiety over the time it takes to get a diagnosis. Obviously, ten years is far too long, but conversely the answer is not to demand a two-week pathway. The ticking clock, chronic pain and fear makes any form of waiting hard to tolerate,

> but if we remember that pain is not proportionate to disease activity (first reassuring flag) and that the threat to our life is not imminent. The reassuring flags can provide some comfort through the wait while the GP follows a medically constructed plan of action.

YOUR FIRST GP VISIT

It is safe to say that the first time a woman goes to the GP complaining of painful or heavy periods is unlikely to be the time she will hear the word 'endometriosis'. Knowing what I know now, I ask myself – should it be? I am not sure, but if I was still practising clinically, I might not always make a woman aware of the condition from the *first* encounter. But I do think the basic understanding and awareness of reproductive health should be taught to all women within schools, and conditions like endometriosis should be covered.

Remember that up to 90 per cent of women will have painful periods during their reproductive years, but only 10 per cent will go on to be diagnosed with endometriosis. It would be very alarmist, bordering inappropriate to put the fear of this incurable disease into every woman who visits their doctor complaining of painful periods.

The majority of women visiting their GP with painful periods *will not have* endometriosis. But what *should* happen is something we doctors call 'safety netting'. Doctors should always safety net before letting a patient leave. This means outlining a plan to follow if things change or don't improve. Encourage patients to *come back* if things get worse or don't improve. This is because *we as doctors know* that there could always be the possibility of other underlying conditions.

It would be inappropriate to always list the things it *could be* in those early encounters because a patient would immediately wonder why a doctor has brought up a specific disease. Hence why the first presentation of period pain shouldn't necessarily warrant a discussion about all the potential causes; it will often be misplaced, cause unnecessary anxiety and most women's symptoms will respond to those early treatments offered.

Your medical history

Having a clear way of communicating with your GP will help smooth the process so that you can help your GP to help you. While tracking your symptoms is unlikely to speed up the diagnosis time, it can help you to recognize a pattern and whether they are cyclical and give you a starting point for opening a discussion with your GP. The best communication tool I can suggest is the ICE method of communication (see page 253). Sometimes less is more when tracking symptoms: what the symptoms are, how bad and how often. Below is what the GP needs to know:

SYMPTOM	PRESENT YES/NO	WHEN IN YOUR CYCLE
General pain		
Pain outside of the pelvis		
Pain or blood passing stools (poo)		
Pain or blood passing urine		
Pain during sex		
Pain after sex		
Flooding		
Passing clots		
Bleeding in-between periods		
Tiredness		

Mood symptoms		
Difficulty trying to conceive		
Miscarriages		
Fevers		
Other symptoms		

At your appointment, the GP will go through your history with you. They will ask about your symptoms and explore them in more detail (how long, where, checking for other symptoms that may never have occurred to you). They will then ask about the visible signs of disease you may not have noticed (see page 103). They may even ask about family history – e.g. have any of the women in your family had endometriosis? – as this can raise the likelihood of you having it.

The examination

The taking of your medical history should be followed by an examination. I know this doesn't always happen, but it should and the ten commandments of the medical system (i.e. the NICE guidelines) state that an examination is needed. Your doctor will more often than not be unlikely to find anything conclusive (i.e. the doctor will not see or feel obvious visible signs or changes on the surface of your body). Most women with endometriosis will have no obvious visible signs when being examined. But the doctor is not just examining you for suspected endometriosis, they are also checking for other potential causes for your symptoms.

An examination may not just be the doctor feeling your stomach – they may want to do a vaginal/internal examination. These examinations are to feel if there are any lumps/bumps/masses where they shouldn't be (again looking for all potential causes, not just endometriosis). A healthy, non-pregnant uterus should sit easily in a position that *can't* be felt. Conditions like fibroids (see page 185), adenomyosis (see page 201) and some others make the uterus enlarged or irregular, which can make it palpable (easily felt) through the stomach wall.

An internal examination can involve the doctor placing one hand on the stomach while two fingers of the other hand are inserted into the vagina and positioned to put pressure on the cervix, pushing the uterus upward so it's easier to feel. This is a very intimate examination, and a chaperone should always be offered if you have attended the appointment alone. It is always okay to ask that a female doctor perform this examination, even if that means rebooking another appointment when one is available.

NEXT STEPS

Even if the doctor agrees that you may have endometriosis, the next step will not necessarily be to immediately refer you to a specialist. What happens next is a pathway of investigations while simultaneously trying different treatment options (medications or methods to relieve symptoms).

For the many different potential causes of painful periods (including adenomyosis and fibroids – see pages 201 and 185) there is a common approach of treatment and investigations. This is a reassuring flag: that while the underlying cause might not yet be known, the majority of the likely causes will respond to the same initial treatments, allowing the GP to begin treatments with confidence that they are covering multiple bases. These treatments would be the same even if (hypothetically) you had a laparoscopy the same day to confirm the diagnosis – the treatments would still start at the same point if following the guidelines.

Painkillers

Before rushing to do a scan, the first step for a GP is to offer pain relief: paracetamol and NSAIDS (non-steroidal anti-inflammatories) such as ibuprofen, naproxen and diclofenac. We tend to assume that paracetamol won't be effective, but it's actually a very good painkiller, especially if taken regularly, and is one of the safest available. I know from experience as a doctor that many people who complain their painkillers aren't working are taking all the stronger ones and seem to skip the basics, seeing them as too trivial to bother with. But it's like a cocktail – paracetamol is the ice. It still needs to go in there even if it doesn't seem as fancy and important as the 'good stuff'.

Why are women offered basic painkillers as the first steps? Because for many women this will be enough. A proportion of these women who don't have underlying conditions, and even those who do, will likely respond well to this first step. The advice to take over-the-counter pain relief is not your GP being dismissive; it is avoiding putting unnecessary strain on resources that may not be needed. With no cure available for endometriosis, the goal of any management options is pain reduction and fertility preservation.

But this is where we need to consider safety netting. If these first line painkillers aren't working, how long should you try them before going back to your GP? If there's really no response within a month or two (or things are getting much worse), book another appointment. If you respond well for even a year or two, but then things change – go back. Repeat your ICE (see page 253).

Hormone treatment

Depending on the examination and the severity of the symptoms, the next step is likely to be trialling a type of hormone treatment (the contraceptive pill, either combined or progesterone-only, see pages 152–9) to help with the pain. Depending on symptoms, for women with low risk or no signs of severe disease it's reasonable for the GP to not immediately arrange a scan. What is needed at this stage is communication that you're now starting a hormone treatment for dysmenorrhoea – and the potential implications of this. An explanation that if things get worse or your body isn't responding to treatment that you may have a suspected underlying condition such as endometriosis. For some women even with endometriosis, this step may be enough and the contraceptive pill could manage the symptoms adequately for many years. But making sure that the conversation is had is key – so that women know if there is a potential for underlying endometriosis what this means for fertility and potential progression of disease when they come off the pill.

Blood tests

Blood tests are not always needed as there is no blood test for endometriosis at the time of writing (although I am confident there will eventually be a method of profiling inflammatory response and other markers). If there is a degree of significantly heavy or ongoing bleeding the GP might test for anaemia, or if there are suggestions of something else going on then blood tests might be arranged, but don't be affronted if you are not offered a blood test.

Imaging

It's important to understand that a negative scan (a scan that says 'nothing seen') does not necessarily mean there is no endometriosis present. Endometriosis is incredibly difficult to diagnose. It is a disease happening at a small cellular level, with the symptoms disproportionate to its size and through a process not easily visible on most scans. Furthermore, endometriosis (in the rare occasions it does appear on a scan) can often only be recognized by a specialist who knows what to look for.

> A negative scan does not mean there is no endometriosis present and cannot rule out the diagnosis, but a positive scan can confirm the diagnosis. In the event of a negative scan, further investigation by way of a laparoscopy may be needed.
>
> You may be wondering why, if scans are not brilliant at detecting endometriosis, we are offered them at all? The simple answer is because some scans, particularly if done by the right people, *can* detect endometriosis, thus giving a diagnosis without the need for surgery. In addition, scans are useful for detecting adhesions, adenomyosis, fibroids, large endometriomas and cancers, which may warrant an urgent referral. Remember endometriosis is not the only potential cause of pain and heavy bleeding, so imaging can be useful for ruling out cancer or alternative diagnoses.

Ultrasound

The first type of scan a GP is likely to arrange is an ultrasound (USS), either over the tummy (TAUS/transabdominal ultrasound) or via the vagina (TVUS/transvaginal ultrasound). An ultrasound is a relatively quick scan for the GP to arrange and doesn't require referral to a specialist consultant.

An ultrasound that goes over the tummy (much the same as done for a pregnancy ultrasound) can be effective to a degree, but often the person doing the scan (radiographer) will want to do an *internal* ultrasound by inserting a probe inside the vagina. This takes a focal point on the probe to look very closely in and around the uterus and up close to the ovaries by getting as close to the cervix and surrounding area. It can be a little uncomfortable, and sometimes even alarming as the clinician covers the probe – which essentially looks like a vibrator attached to a TV monitor – in a condom and lubrication. Remember that you can always have a chaperone present (if you've attended the appointment alone you can ask for a chaperone), it's over very quickly and can be helpful to identify any urgent problems which need addressing.

If you aren't offered an ultrasound in your pathway from 'suspected' to 'confirmed' endometriosis, this isn't because you're being overlooked or not given the best care. The need for this step is very much a patient-by-patient decision made by the GP, guided by the NICE guidelines.

MRI

The imaging type best suited to identifying endometriosis is an MRI, but again the chance of diagnosis using this method is increased if the scan is carried out by an endometriosis/gynaecology specialist radiologist.

An MRI machine is a long tube where you lie on a bed and slide into the machine. It can be quite claustrophobic and the noise of the magnets rotating is very loud, meaning that some patients are anxious about this type of scan. However, it's usually over within 30–45 minutes and not everyone needs their heads to go into the scanner. You will usually be offered headphones to listen to music to help you stay as calm and relaxed as possible.

An MRI can sometimes help identify adhesions and advanced disease, particularly bowel or bladder involvement. Sometimes the gynaecology surgeon will arrange an MRI prior to a laparoscopy (see below), not so much to help the diagnosis but to get an understanding of what to expect during surgery. If the MRI detects that there is extensive and obvious bowel involvement, the surgical team can plan for the right specialists to be present in the surgery.

Previously it was stated that the 'gold standard' way of diagnosing endometriosis was through a laparoscopy; however, this is no longer the case as advances in MRI imaging and specialist radiologist training have improved.

Laparoscopy

A laparoscopy is often considered to be a tool for treatment, but it is actually one of the best diagnostic methods for endometriosis. Up until a few years ago a laparoscopy was considered the main way of diagnosing endometriosis, but as it is a high-risk, invasive procedure it's not an easy process for a patient. A laparoscopy allows a surgeon to look directly into the abdomen in real time to see what the anatomy looks like, any disease activity and take biopsies if needed.

During a laparoscopy, three small holes are made in the stomach for the surgeon to insert three probes. These probes can inflate the stomach with air like a balloon to make it easy to move around and view the organs. One of the probes has a camera and a light to project what it is pointing at onto a screen. The others have tools the surgeon can use to cut and move things out of the way to navigate around the organs.

This method of surgery is much safer than a laparotomy, which involves opening the entire abdomen up with a larger incision (cut). Because a laparoscopy doesn't require cutting the entire abdominal muscles, it is quicker to recover from and carries less surgical risk of infection and other complications.

The purpose of a diagnostic laparoscopy is to look at what is happening to the organs to aid a diagnosis. It's considered the ultimate way to diagnose endometriosis. Whereas a normal MRI or USS does not rule out a diagnosis of endometriosis, if a laparoscopy shows no signs of endometriosis, this usually means there isn't any.

Most of the time, a surgeon will manage to see the visible endometriotic lesions or signs or scarring or adhesions. The surgeon can (and often will) also do biopsies. A biopsy means taking a small cutting of the tissue that they suspect is the endometriosis, and then another doctor (pathologist) will look at this tissue under a microscope to check that the cells are indeed endometriotic. The surgeon can give the diagnosis if they see endometriosis, and the biopsy is often there for double confirmation, as well as confirming the damaged tissue is nothing more sinister, such as cancer cells. If there is an endometrioma present (this is a large mass on or around an ovary) then they will need to do a biopsy because of the risk of endometriomas becoming malignant.

There are occasions where the endometriosis is not easily visible, particularly if it's a deep, early lesion, or small and not much associated scarring has occurred. Endometriosis specialist surgeons are usually good at spotting these and will know to take biopsies in ambiguous places. Sometimes these can be missed by a gynaecological surgeon who is not a specialist in endometriosis, which is why they are also encouraged to take biopsies which might pick up lesions that are not easily visible.

Waiting for a laparoscopy

Waiting lists for a laparoscopy can be a year or two (in some cases, up to five years). This may seem like a painfully long wait to a patient, particularly a woman who has already had years of tests and investigations. However, there is a system in place within hospitals to ensure clinical urgency is prioritized.

When you are listed for a surgical procedure like a laparoscopy, you are triaged for how soon you need it based on clinical need. Clinical need means the doctors will review the notes and patients with signs suggesting risk of organ damage are put into a faster track compared to those with less urgent symptoms.

If you have been on the waiting list for a while, things are getting worse and you are truly struggling, you can phone the hospital to find out where you are in the waiting list. If this seems far too long and you are really not managing (e.g. unable to manage the pain, which is affecting your ability to work, etc.), your GP can liaise with the hospital and ask to put you onto a more urgent list. While you're waiting it is important to remember to take as much support as you can to enable you to function alongside the pain. It is important to remember that the GP can provide effective treatments and support while you are waiting for the laparoscopy.

My story

A lot of people expect that if a surgeon is putting you through the not-so-easy process of having the surgery, that they will also 'treat' the endometriosis while in there. It can come as a real shock to discover that a surgeon can see something wrong and not touch it, and even delay starting any management. This is exactly what happened to me the first time I had a laparoscopy, which first identified early stages of endometriosis. I was appalled at the time, but I know now that this was, in part, the right decision. This is because the surgeon diagnosing the endometriosis may not be trained with the advanced skills needed to remove the endometriosis disease they find during the laparoscopy. They will therefore need to refer you on to a more specialist surgeon to ensure you receive the best care.

In my case, what I didn't appreciate at the time was had the surgeon tried to treat my endometriosis at that point he would have likely done more harm than good because he wasn't skilled or trained to remove those endometriosis lesions. He was right not to touch them. But what was wrong in my personal situation was that he did not start me on any form of treatment (medication), nor refer me to the right specialist who *could* attempt surgical repair. He discharged me with a diagnosis and no treatment plan whatsoever. That was wrong. Suffice to say it is not always inappropriate for a surgeon to do a laparoscopy for the purpose of diagnosing without the intention to treat at the same time. But there should be a plan moving on from the diagnosis for how you will be managed thereafter and who should care for you moving forwards.

THE LONG WAIT

Waiting ten years for a diagnosis feels appalling, but this is a disease which manifests slowly and has elusive symptoms that are not related to periods, such as bowel cramps and joint pains. It is also important to remember that the process of diagnosing endometriosis shouldn't happen without the GP providing supportive treatment at the same time. Many of these women going for years and years without a diagnosis (as the headlines suggest) are not being left without treatment. They may sometimes be left without understanding, counselling or support, but they are not always left without treatment.

Patience is key, as is understanding that the offer of painkillers and the contraceptive pill are not a tool to 'fob you off'. The slow process of diagnosis is not necessarily neglecting the urgency that you might feel there *should be* because of how much pain you are suffering. It is this oversight in communication between doctors and patients that I fear leads to a breakdown in trust, rise in frustration and disengagement with medications.

Women are in a lot of pain, their bodies are screaming that something is wrong, but they have been given the pill and told to wait six months for an MRI. This is actually a reasonable step for most women and, as difficult as it may be, we must trust the process (when the process is done properly, of course).

Suspected endometriosis: an interim diagnosis

Often, while waiting for the official confirmation of the presence or absence of endometriosis, the term 'suspected endometriosis' will be used. This alerts all medical professionals that you have all the symptoms for, and are being treated for, suspected endometriosis and are essentially waiting for the official confirmation.

Because endometriosis is not an easy or quick disease to diagnose, the way you present as a patient (your signs or symptoms) can often be evidence enough for a GP to begin treatment. They can do this while arranging the scans and any referrals. This diagnosis will eventually be turned into a 'confirmed endometriosis' or, for a small minority, '*not* endometriosis'; for the latter the road to exploring other explanations begins.

Being on this pathway of 'suspected' allows for the care and support to be given, while allowing for the time it takes for the official confirmation to be reached (another reassuring flag). At this point your GP will likely decide whether to refer you to secondary care (such as a gynaecologist), but the timing for being referred to a specialist is not set in stone. There is no definitive point at which a GP needs to refer and this very much depends on the individual patient. Similarly, depending on what the symptoms and signs are suggesting, the GP has the option of referring to gynaecology in general, or an endometriosis specialist (secondary or tertiary care).

The guidelines have been established in an attempt to separate the pathways so that women who have suspected milder disease are referred to general gynaecology, whereas those with more advanced disease are referred to the specialists. The demand on resources would be overwhelming and there simply is not the facility for the limited number of endometriosis specialists to see *all* the suspected endometriosis patients.

When you consider the fact that symptoms do not reflect size and severity of underlying disease, you could see how it is inevitable that some women find themselves with a general gynaecologist who is not trained to deal with stage three or four disease. This does not mean the system is entirely flawed – a large proportion of women with mild-moderate disease will be properly and well managed by the routine gynaecology pathway and a general gynaecologist surgeon.

The reasons for being referred straight to an endometriosis specialist are if the GP suspects (or it is found on imaging) an endometrioma (see page 134), deep endometriosis with bowel or bladder involvement or endometriosis outside of the pelvic area. If a diagnostic laparoscopy identifies advanced disease while under the routine pathway, then the patient is usually referred on to a more specialist endometriosis surgeon.

It's important to remember that GPs do not always need to refer every single suspected endometriosis case to a hospital specialist (secondary or tertiary). If the patient's symptoms are mild a scan may not necessarily be done. The GP can in this instance treat a woman for *suspected endometriosis* more than adequately with the management options available to them – and if all is well, why burden the hospital system? A large proportion of women *will* respond well to treatment. The caveat here being that there is open communication with the patient so they are aware of this. Full autonomy means being fully informed of the situation.

Another potential situation is that the GP may start treatment and arrange some scans, and if at any point more severe disease is suggested, either from symptoms or a scan, then they will refer appropriately. This could be one to two years into the process. This is why, for endometriosis, taking several years for a diagnosis is not wholly inappropriate.

A typical scenario

Imagine this commonly occurring scenario: a woman first presents in her early twenties with painful periods. The GP rightly starts her on an oral contraceptive pill. It may or may not be even documented in her notes as being for suspected endometriosis, but it will be documented as dysmenorrhoea (painful periods). *This is the point where early discussions should be had to warn a woman of the potential other causes for the painful periods, such as endometriosis, so that she can have an awareness of her own body and be vigilant over time if anything changes.*

The woman continues for two to three years managing well and no complaints. She comes off the pill to begin trying for a baby. The pain comes back, worse than before. The GP arranges an ultrasound, which is normal. The woman is managing well on new pain relief offered and is still trying to get pregnant.

In this instance the woman may or may not have endometriosis. It might be that over the next two years she continues to have difficulty getting pregnant, the pain is getting worse and at this point the GP refers to gynaecology – she receives her diagnosis of endometriosis another year later after a laparoscopy confirms the disease. Her diagnosis was 'technically' six years after her first presentation to the GP with painful periods – but was this the result of neglect by the system? No: everyone was following a pathway that was reasonable and in response in the moment to the patient's needs. This hypothetical patient absolutely might have had endometriosis at that first presentation, but the management for this would have been exactly the same had she had the laparoscopy the first time she saw the GP, being treated with oral hormone tablets to help her symptoms. As the symptoms progressed, the GP responded accordingly.

This is a common scenario and the pathway is, in fact, reasonable. What does need to change is that any woman being treated or scanned for a suspected diagnosis or for primary dysmenorrhoea needs to know so that she is informed and aware to be vigilant in case things change or progress, meaning the diagnosis or speed of investigations needs to be changed. Part of the reason I fear for the lengthy diagnosis time is that so many women are prescribed the contraceptive pill for dysmenorrhoea without it being clear whether this is to treat the symptoms of primary dysmenorrhoea or suspected secondary dysmenorrhoea. As a result, these women continue for many years totally unaware of the need to be keeping an eye for other symptoms suggesting endometriosis (bowel pain, pain during sex, etc.). If they were simply given this information right at the start of being managed for painful periods, so many could potentially reach their diagnosis much earlier.

SUSPECTED TO CONFIRMED

Hearing the words 'yes you have endometriosis' can be a real mixed bag of emotions. For some it can feel like a long-awaited gift providing access to vindication, support, treatment and understanding. For others it may reinforce a lot of uncertainty and create new anxiety over what the future looks like for pain, infertility and future surgeries. The truth is that the disease is incurable, and with any life-changing diagnosis like this there comes a grief response, called disenfranchised grief (see page 248).

By the time you get a diagnosis of endometriosis you may have been receiving treatment for months if not years. What might change now is that the surgeon may have a better idea as to what stage your endometriosis is and what the longer-term management plan is (see pages 145–70).

Post-surgery

When you wake up from the surgery and are told the outcome of your laparoscopy, quite often the surgeon is doing their round to check in on you while you are still groggy from the anaesthetic and haven't had your first bite of hospital toast yet. I have always found this frustrating as a patient – having a really important conversation at a time when you're not fully lucid is not ideal, and chances are you won't see the consultant again for a few weeks or months until clinic, if at all.

To counter this, have your questions already prepared and take a pen and paper if needed, or ask the nurse to note down what is said. They will likely add these details to your discharge notes but be prepared for a quick conversation.

The surgeon will likely briefly cover the following key outcomes from the surgery (and if not offered by the surgeon, key points for you to ask):

- Endometriosis: confirmed diagnosis or not present (and what next in terms of ongoing care).
- Staging: not every surgeon likes to discuss staging with patients because it isn't reflective of symptom severity but it is important to know (see page 96).
- Bowel or bladder involvement and, if so, how bad and what next.
- Are the ovaries damaged, if there is an endometrioma present, and if so, were biopsies taken.
- Fallopian tubes: whether these were damaged at all or appear open (patent), which is important for fertility.
- If they attempted to remove any of the plaques/disease.

The next part of the conversation needs to be: what are the next steps? Is the surgeon planning on another procedure to go back in and remove the endometriosis? Are they planning on inducing menopause through medication for a short time? Do you need to change what type of hormone treatments you are on? If you are told you have stage three or four disease, ask whether you are being referred to an endometriosis specialist surgeon.

If it is stage one or two, the next thing to ask is are they keeping you under their care for follow up or discharging you back to the GP? *If they are keeping you under their care, then you will likely have access to an endometriosis specialist nurse: ask for their number.*

It has likely been a long road to get to this point, and the post-surgery time can present a surreal anti-climax, a wave of relief or switching between several emotions. Alongside this you need to heal and take time to process the news. At this point it is often useful to revisit the resources, learn more about what this news means and how best to equip yourself for what is probably a lifelong diagnosis (if confirmed).

Even though endometriosis is incurable this doesn't mean you will have pain or other problems at their current severity for your entire life. There are a lot of women who find a place of 'getting on top' of the disease; some even find a place of being pain free. The path is uncertain, though, and how you navigate what lies ahead needs to be a two-way process involving your team *and you*. Taking confidence in your right to autonomy in the choices about your care can come with equipping yourself with the right knowledge

IF IT'S NOT ENDOMETRIOSIS

Imagine having problematic periods for many years. You are then under the umbrella of 'suspected endometriosis' for a few more years and finally feel like there are answers, which in turn offers hope. For a diagnosis suggests a treatment plan, and something for the team around you to understand why you are struggling the way you are. For some people this may have been the first operation you've ever had, which is (in itself) daunting and a major life event. And then you wake up from surgery to be told there is no endometriosis. In a game of snakes and ladders, you were one step from the finish line and landed on a snake you didn't know was there and are right back to square one.

First – take a pause. Heal. You have just undergone a surgical procedure after months, if not years, of waiting and uncertainty. Hormones are all over the place, there is still the ongoing pain and instead of an answer you now face more uncertainty and the realization you are no further forward. Take a pause. Feel all the feels, those emotions are entirely valid and justified. Sit in them. Communicate and share them with those around you and find support in communities who understand.

It can be devastating. Again, the irony of being disappointed to *not* have an incurable disease may seem beyond comprehension to some. But not to a person who has got to the point of needing that laparoscopy and going through the long arduous process of scans, waiting and pain.

One would hope at this point a good GP would step in to catch you mid-fall and reassure that they will still explore other options and remind you that for many women, primary dysmenorrhoea is a diagnosis and that there is still support available.

There are other causes for the pain which wouldn't necessarily show up on the laparoscopy and so it is always crucial to remember that you know your body. If there are still symptoms and issues, there are still things to be explored between you and your GP: turn to Chapter 13 on page 245 to help guide you through times of uncertainty. It is also important to know that for a very small minority of women, particularly if the diagnostic laparoscopy was done by a gynaecologist not particularly specialized in endometriosis, small/low-level disease can be missed. More specialist surgeons are trained and familiar with taking biopsies to avoid missing small disease plaques. In some instances, it is possible to ask whether a second opinion from a specialist is worth exploring.

My story

Would an earlier diagnosis have changed the outcome for me?

I am now more than 20 years into my life with painful, dysfunctional periods. My endometriosis diagnosis was about eight years ago, my hysterectomy was four years ago, and I am still facing more surgeries for advanced disease that just will not budge despite having all my reproductive organs (including my cervix) removed. There was a time I truly felt my degree of disability would have been different had I been 'managed better' earlier on.

However, I do believe the outcome would have been the same. Maybe at a different time of life, maybe to a different extent. The journey would have been different for sure, but I must acknowledge that my dysfunctional immune system was always going to react the way it did to the endometriosis, and that ultimately, I was always going to need a hysterectomy.

> When and how that happened may have been different, and the needless challenges along the way could have been avoided. But to sit here knowing what I know now about the body's responsibility for this disease and how it behaves – I was likely always destined to have advanced disease. There could have been all the right services, all the right clinicians along the way – but the truth is my body was doing what it was going to do and the way it responded to the disease could not have been changed. In the absence of a cure for endometriosis, I recognize that I was likely always going to need a hysterectomy. A hysterectomy and advanced disease are not, despite how it is depicted sometimes on social media, the result of poor management.

CHAPTER SUMMARY

Understanding the complexities of how endometriosis manifests and presents will help to lay the foundations for why it is so difficult to diagnose. The onset of symptoms with endometriosis is not sudden and our society's historical and cultural attitudes to labelling painful periods as 'normal' has contributed to this lengthy time for a diagnosis. We aren't always equipped with the right knowledge to recognize these symptoms ourselves, let alone know when to seek help to identify the underlying cause.

Having an appreciation and awareness of the fact that many women with painful periods have primary dysmenorrhoea and will respond well to hormone treatments – and that these hormone treatments are also the early interventional approaches for endometriosis itself – should hopefully restore some trust and relieve anxiety. When a suspicion of having endometriosis arises, the immediate reaction for wanting intervention, surgery and specialist referral is understandable, but medical urgency isn't always warranted. This is not always a dismissal, but a reasonable medical approach.

I hope that the outline of how the system works – the process from 'suspected' to 'confirmed' diagnosis – will offer some reassurance that along this journey you are not without support. Treatment begins alongside this journey and while the wait can feel agonizing, it is not without tools to regain quality of life along the way.

Key takeaways

- Nine out of ten women have painful periods (dysmenorrhoea), but the reality is that only one in ten will be diagnosed with endometriosis. Both are a diagnosis, both have options for support, and treatment for both in the early stages have a strong overlap. Therefore, if early approaches by the GP are to start treatment to cover both, this isn't necessarily dismissal or failure to respond; it is a measured approach in recognition of probability, risk and presenting symptoms.
- Specialist MRI scans and radiologists can sometimes detect endometriosis, with a positive scan result to confirm a diagnosis. However, a negative ultrasound or MRI does not rule out an endometriosis diagnosis. The definitive way to diagnose is through a surgical procedure (laparoscopy) in which a specialist surgeon looks directly within the pelvis to see visible endometriosis and takes biopsies if needed for further confirmation.
- The process and pathway for diagnosis can be lengthy, but the wait is not without treatment options. Medication treatments (hormone and non-hormone-based) do and should begin alongside the diagnosis pathway.

CHAPTER 7:
ENDOMETRIOSIS MANAGEMENT

A BROAD APPROACH

I would love to say that there is a step ladder approach to treating endometriosis, as there is for many other conditions, where you would try a first line treatment and then if it fails, you would move on to the next. Inevitably, with a disease as unpredictable and inconsistent as endometriosis, our approach to management needs is broad to reflect your overarching goals.

Before embarking on a treatment plan it's important to have a good understanding of what your personal goals for treatment are. Discussing this with your GP or gynaecologist is key. We know that endometriosis *has no cure* so considering what you and the team are hoping to achieve in terms of pain management and fertility preservation is paramount.

This is because a large proportion of the medications used to treat the pain of endometriosis are hormone based which, through their action, induce a contraceptive state. (Fertility is covered in more depth in Chapter 8 on pages 171–184). When targeting pain as your main goal, knowing now that pain is not proportionate to disease activity needs to be considered. Similarly, recognizing that using hormone treatments to improve pain is not necessarily 'masking' something more serious. Had I known this earlier on in my own journey I would have been a lot more compliant with the pain relief medications offered and consequently suffered a lot less! I suffered for years with avoidable pain, anxiety and a feeling of being 'fobbed off' – all because the crucial information I'm presenting here wasn't presented to me.

UNDERSTANDING THE GOALS OF MANAGEMENT

It took me a long time to find a combination of treatments that worked for me in managing my endometriosis. I have reflected on why I found it so difficult to make sense of the treatments being offered, while wrestling with my own reluctance to engage with some options, as well as my repeated failures to find anything that worked. Eventually, I realized what was missing: an understanding of what the *aim* of management *actually* is. The answer is probably not what you are expecting.

After years of engaging with women both as a doctor and as an advocate and hearing countless familiar stories, I recognized that if I, as a doctor, had missed the point, then I was surely not alone. What almost everyone wants to know when they receive a diagnosis (of any kind) is: *how do I get rid of it?* If it turns out that the condition cannot be eradicated, the next question is often: *will it kill me?*

Although endometriosis cannot be cured or eradicated fully from the body, it is not life-threatening. The good news is that it should not shorten your life; the difficult reality is that its incurable nature often leaves you facing a chronic disease that can, and for many does, deeply impact your quality of life.

But there is hope. From my research, I believe that the quality of life for women with endometriosis could be mitigated quite significantly. How? By better understanding the purpose of treatments – engaging with the process would likely improve people's experiences.

Many women manage to find a treatment regime that works for them: keeping their pain relatively well controlled, regaining their quality of life and learning to live a life that isn't defined or controlled by their disease. To do this, you need to be fully equipped and informed with the tools to approach the disease's management.

From my personal and professional experience, I believe that many women who are struggling with their disease and feeling that it's 'out of control' or find themselves at a point of desperation face this for two main reasons:

1. **Women are not established on the right management plan *for them*.** If a patient struggles with side effects, then their compliance (commitment to treatment) will likely decline, pulling them further away from where they want to be in terms of disease management and quality of life. Hormonal treatments are often the first port of call, but intolerance to these, especially due to the impact they can have on mental wellbeing, is often a big factor in compliance. Improved compliance can be achieved by a better dialogue between patient and doctor about which hormones are involved in each treatment, and by patients being empowered through knowledge and guidance to have a self-awareness of which hormones they are more sensitive to.
2. **Women don't understand the aims of management**, and so their compliance is poor, to the detriment of their own health. This is especially true for treatments that predominantly aim to reduce pain and improve quality of life as they don't target the physical spread of disease.

Only in the last few years have I finally understood what the aims of management truly are for me; once I had that lightbulb moment it changed the way I viewed my own treatment options. It transformed the way I tolerated certain side effects and immediately put an end to my reluctance at taking pain relief (which I initially worried was just going to mask pain that I perceived as a genuine warning siren).

When you fully understand what the aim of a treatment is and what is happening, you are far more likely to respond and engage. When we have a realistic expectation of the future it can change everything. But why do these two obstacles affect so many people?

The obstacles to effective management

First, not enough doctors are trained extensively in endometriosis, as there simply isn't the time, resources or prioritization. Consequently, many doctors follow what they believe to be a standard pathway of treatment without the full understanding of how to use treatment options or adapt them to the patient. For many conditions in medicine there is a singular, clear pathway – a ladder of treatment options where if one doesn't work, you move to the next. But unfortunately, this doesn't work for endometriosis.

The disease is not the same for everyone, and there is no 'one size fits all' treatment plan, least of all a stepwise approach. As discussed on page 154, two women could present with the same disease picture (either in physical form or in symptom form, bearing in mind that symptoms do not always correlate with physical findings), but what helps one may not necessarily help the other.

Which leads to the next problem with management plans: women's understanding of the treatments. Endometriosis cannot be cured and no treatment is given with this intention. This is something that many patients are not aware of. Palliative care, contrary to popular misunderstanding, is an area of medicine that provides supportive care by helping patients live as well as possible for as long as possible. Treatment options for endometriosis are just this: aimed at holding back the disease's spread, preventing or delaying organ damage, minimizing pain and preserving or attaining fertility (this last part is very much patient led).

The most important aspect patients need to be aware of is that the aim of treatments is entirely symptom management. No treatment will eradicate the disease or reverse it. Surgical options attempt to remove plaques as best as possible, but the disease can – and often does – re-grow. I see too many times patients hearing the word 'treatment' and presuming it means 'cure'. Treatments are methods of managing disease or reducing symptoms and are not synonymous with cures for disease. Ideally when discussing treatment options, the doctors should explain what the intention of any treatment is: to cure or to improve quality of life. In endometriosis, any treatment offered is purely to improve quality of life. There is no cure.

The second aspect of understanding the mechanisms of hormone treatments is appreciating what is happening at a disease level. This is the part that so many women misunderstand. I absolutely fell into this category and given that I am medically trained, it should testify to how poorly understood and communicated this disease is.

For years I struggled – and at times outright refused – to take certain painkillers or hormone treatments because I felt I was being fobbed off. This was despite being in a huge amount of pain. That survival mechanism within me was raising alarm bells incessantly: something was wrong, my organs must be being ripped to shreds given the amount of pain I was in. I could not understand why the studies on different treatments were only monitoring patients' responses to pain as a measure of how good a treatment option was. Why was no one checking response in terms of the physical size of the plaques?

As a result, I didn't want to take painkillers and mask my pain – I was genuinely terrified that by masking the pain, I was risking my life. After years of frustration, I had an appointment where I was again told to take stronger painkillers, and something inside me snapped. How was I being fobbed off again after all these years? Then the penny dropped. Through a deep dive into physiology books, I realized something that changed everything. I finally understood two things:

1. **The pain is not proportionate to disease activity.** If someone has visually assessed your insides (through MRI or laparoscopy) and confirmed that you are not in immediate danger, then it is entirely appropriate to silence those overactive pain receptors by taking pain relief. Their signals – akin to tsunami-level warnings – are misfiring. This is not like having a heart attack and being told to take paracetamol – even if the level of pain you are in is making you feel that your level of disease must be severe.
2. **You are never going to get rid of the disease.** Hence why the success of a hormone treatment is not measured by the physical activity of the disease but by how much quality of life a woman regains while on it.

MEDICATION VERSUS SURGERY

There are two approaches to tackling endometriosis: medication and surgery. In the absence of a cure, the balance of risk and benefit of these two approaches needs to be considered.

It's best to decide on your priorities early on, although this may change over time. Is your biggest grievance pain and disruption to quality of life? Is it symptoms associated with advanced disease, such as bowel disruption? Or is it fertility?

Bearing in mind that treatments for endometriosis are not aimed at curing the disease but at managing pain and fertility, there are important questions every woman needs to ask when approaching treatment options:

> *What is my goal for treatment? Is it to get on top of the pain or is it fertility? And if fertility is the goal, am I wanting to conceive now or do I have time to manage the disease first to improve my chances?*

The reason these questions are important is because the majority of medication-centred treatments to manage pain are hormone based, which means that by proxy they are also a form of contraceptive. Knowing what your primary focus is (pain or fertility) greatly influences what treatments are *right for you*.

Some treatment options can buy time, in that they can delay the need for surgery, preserve organ function or limit damage to the ovaries. If you aren't sure what the right option is for you, you can discuss this with your doctor.

It's also worth noting that *you don't need to be under a gynaecologist to receive treatment for endometriosis*. Whether you are still waiting for a laparoscopy or your GP is treating you for suspected endometriosis, there are multiple options available in primary care to support your symptoms. Many women feel they need to be referred immediately to a specialist. But if the disease can be controlled by a GP then it's a path that can work well, and is far more accessible. To ensure the best care, I recommend asking at your practice if there is a GP with a special interest in gynaecological health. You can do this at any point in your journey to diagnosis and beyond.

PAIN MEDICATION

One of the biggest failings I have seen is the lack of adequate pain relief support for women with endometriosis. It is important to reassure women that, in this instance, it is absolutely okay to dampen those pain receptors and tune them out.

Pain relief is managed stepwise (i.e. working through the various options step by step), and it is important to work with doctors to balance side effects and find a regime that comes as close as possible to managing the pain. It isn't like for like, where doctors only prescribe the 'hard stuff' for severe pain and skip the basics. Pain relief is more like a cocktail or a recipe for a cake. You build the components, making them more effective by combining them. It's usual to start with paracetamol and ibuprofen and then assess their effectiveness before trying the next thing. Skipping paracetamol and ibuprofen (if safe for you) is like skipping the flour or butter in a cake recipe; they are essential and can work very well with stronger options.

I always brace when I utter the words 'paracetamol and ibuprofen' to patients because I empathize with how dismissive it can feel for them. When someone is saying their pain is an eight out of ten and you offer what feels like sugary syrup we give to children, it seems disproportionate, inadequate and even offensive. But these medications can be very effective when used correctly. The key thing is: if these aren't working then you *add in* stronger options through discussion with your GP.

Pregnancy

There are non-hormonal pain relief options that are safe to use while trying to conceive, though always discuss this with your doctor to confirm suitability. It is important to always check with your GP or pharmacist if you think you are pregnant as some over-the-counter pain relief options are not safe to use in pregnancy.

A type of pain relief doctors may offer which often lands poorly if not explained well, is antidepressants. I must caveat here: yes, some doctors regrettably prescribe these inappropriately, implying the pain is psychological. That is not what I am referring to here. Certain antidepressants also target specific neuroreceptors and have an analgesic effect and in this context they are prescribed for pain relief, not for mood. If you are offered this option by your doctor, it's worth asking if they have prescribed antidepressants for pain relief or for mood. If it is that the GP is using an antidepressant that is also a licensed analgesic, discuss how this can affect your mood and other side effects. Some antidepressants are given at a different dose when used for pain relief purposes, so shouldn't cause any changes in mood.

Beyond prescribed painkillers, other supportive approaches that can help include heat packs, TENS machines, hot baths and cannabidiol (CBD) remedies – but it is always important to check which options are suitable if there is a chance of pregnancy. I went through countless lavender-scented microwave beanbags over the years – they became like a ragged, over-loved bear that followed me around the house. At work, I often used heat packs designed for muscle pain under my scrubs. Do be careful of burns, though; I have seen women so desperate for relief that they ignored the pain of burning skin. If you reach that level of desperation, it is time to revisit your GP for other options.

HORMONAL TREATMENTS

A disease driven by hormones is inevitably approached with treatments that aim to change their balance – often by adding in more hormones, which can be confusing.

Endometriosis is a steroid-dependent disease, meaning the plaques rely on and are stimulated to grow by oestrogen. As a result, treatments have focused on manipulating both oestrogen and progesterone. By reducing oestrogen, the aim is to stop endometrial tissue from growing and lessen the sensitivity of those hyper-reactive, oestrogen-sensitive pain receptors. Meanwhile, raising progesterone should further thin the endometrium and shrink plaques. This is a tricky balancing act which is patient-dependent in terms of tolerance to these hormonal shifts.

It may seem counterintuitive that some hormone treatments will contain oestrogen when the ultimate goal is to reduce it, but removing oestrogen altogether is not ideal because this induces a menopausal state and affects the body as a whole, and not just menstruation. Oestrogen is vital not just for reproduction but for bone, tissue and whole-body health so we don't want to remove it altogether or induce menopause for all women with endometriosis. The absence of oestrogen can 'age' the body quickly, and in younger women especially this carries significant risk of osteoporosis as well as significantly increasing the risk of cardiovascular disease later in life.

To offset this, where treatments deplete natural oestrogen levels to such a degree, some regimens include a small dose of added oestrogen for bone protection. Some treatments also have a limit on how long they can be used.

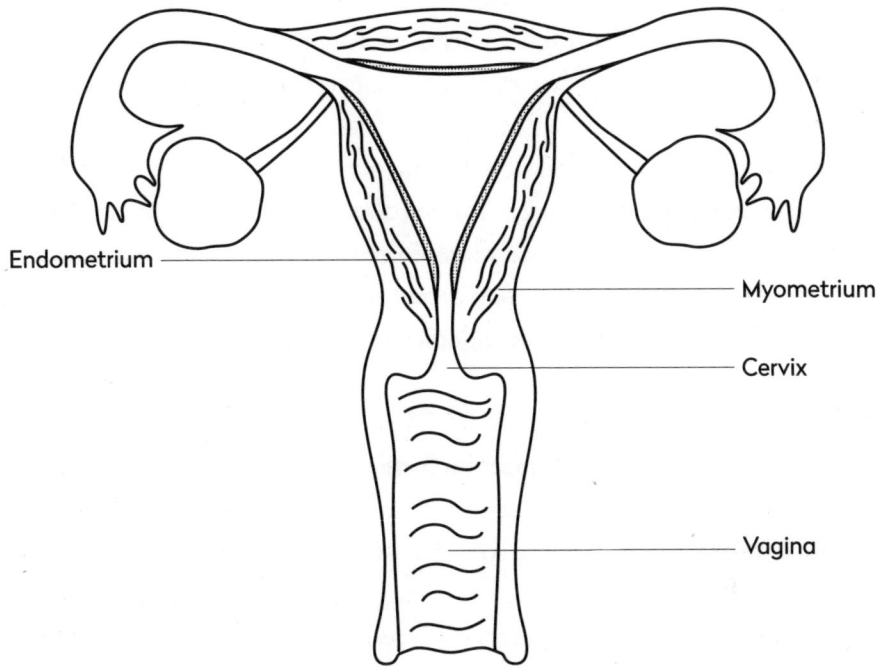

Uterus with thin endometrium

How hormone treatments work

Hormone treatments work by:

- **Lowering oestrogen**, which reduces disease activity and pain.
- **Raising progesterone** to thin the endometrium and plaques.
- **Blocking oestrogen activity** to induce chemical menopause.

Hormone treatments do not remove or reverse endometrial plaques. Instead, they put the lesions into a dormant state. This buys you time until you want to become pregnant or reach a natural menopause, or simply slows progression and prevents organ damage.

Some women with particularly aggressive disease will still find that endometriosis grows, albeit more slowly, despite hormone treatment. This is down to the complexity and unpredictability of the disease. One woman may experience significant pain relief with a treatment that does little to halt plaque growth, while another may see reduced disease activity but little change in pain.

Until now, the only medication treatments for endometriosis have been hormone-based, aimed at altering hormone balance to tackle the disease. But we are moving toward treatments that manipulate the immune system to stop the dysregulation, which is an entirely new approach to endometriosis management. I am delighted to see drug trials for endometriosis shifting away from hormone-based options.

Impact on fertility

Because most hormone-based treatments are contraceptive in nature, many women who are actively trying to conceive will understandably dismiss them outright.

Sometimes taking a break from trying to conceive – allowing the body to rest from the inflammation, pain and distress of the disease – can offer emotional and physical reprieve. The emotional stress of trying to conceive is often underappreciated until experienced first-hand: sex becoming a process rather than for pleasure, the monthly torment of waiting for a period and the creeping fear that pregnancy will never happen. The toll on mental health and relationships can be immense.

Side effects

Contraceptive effects are not the only side effects of hormone treatments. The real impact stems from the hormones themselves and how the body responds.

Some women tolerate shifts in oestrogen or progesterone without issue. Others experience side effects that can vary in their severity from person to person: acne, mood changes, anxiety or depression can all occur to varying degrees. These side effects are usually in response to the culprit that is the synthetic form of progesterone – the progestins.

> **Progestogen**
>
> It's worth noting that progesterone is the natural hormone, whereas the artificial form given in treatments is progestogen. Progestins are the individual synthetic types of progestogen, of which different versions exist. Because there are many types of progestins, one may cause unbearable side effects while another is well tolerated. Women aren't always aware of this and so have a bad reaction to one progestogen-only pill and then write them all off without realizing they may tolerate a different one better. Therefore, the knee-jerk response to avoiding progestogen is premature.

Reflecting on your own history with contraception or PMS (premenstrual syndrome) can help identify sensitivities. Are symptoms worse during certain times in your cycle? Or when taking specific contraceptives? This information can guide more personalized choices. It may be that there is one type of progestin you struggle to tolerate, but a different type may be okay.

For me, anything that raised progesterone triggered anxiety and low mood to an unbearable degree. I once assumed hormones in general were the culprit, but later realized progestogen or progesterone, whether natural or synthetic, was my personal nemesis. Similarly, if I'm given too much oestrogen it triggers my pain receptors. It took me a long while to find the balance that worked, and even to this day I struggle with HRT for these reasons.

Hormone types and how they're delivered

Hormone treatments are not all tablet based. Delivery methods vary:

- **Oral tablets**: oestrogen-only, progesterone-only, or combined.
- **Vaginal ring**: slow-release delivery.
- **Implant**: progestogen delivered via a small device under the skin.
- **IUD (intrauterine device, commonly called the coil)**: progestogen released directly within the uterus.
- **Injection**: three-monthly injections of progestogen.

Hormone base	Treatment	Brand name	Drug name	How it's taken	Side effects	How long
OESTROGEN	Combined oral contraceptive pill (COCP)	Microgynon, Rigevidon, Yasmin, Marvelon	Ethinylestradiol + levonorgestrel, Drospirenone/desogestrel	Tablet	Nausea, breast tenderness, mood changes, spotting, increased clotting risk	Daily, continuous
	Combined contraceptive patch	Evra	Ethinylestradiol + norelgestromin	Patch	Skin irritation, breast tenderness, headaches, mood	Weekly patch (continuous or cyclic)
	Vaginal ring	NuvaRing	Ethinylestradiol + etonogestrel	Vagina	Vaginal irritation, discharge, headaches, mood	3 weeks in, 1 week out OR continuous
PROGESTERONE BASED (Progestogen only) *POP is progesterone only pill	Levonorgestrel IUS (LNG-IUS)	Mirena, Kyleena, Levosert, Jaydess	Levonorgestrel	IUD (coil in uterus via vagina)	Irregular bleeding, no periods, cysts, breast tenderness, mood changes	3–8 years
	Desogestrel POP	Cerelle, Cerazette	Desogestrel	Tablet	Irregular bleeding, mood changes, acne, low libido	Daily, continuous
	Norethisterone/levonorgestrel POP	Noriday, Micronor	Norethisterone/Levonorgestrel	Tablet	Breakthrough bleeding, breast tenderness	Daily, continuous

	High-dose norethisterone		Norethisterone	Tablet	Bloating, acne, mood changes, low libido	Daily, cyclical
	Dienogest	Visanne	Dienogest	Tablet	Irregular bleeding, headaches, mood changes	Daily
	Depot injection DMPA	Depo-Provera, Sayana Press	Medroxyprogesterone acetate	IM or SC injection	Weight gain, low mood, no periods	Every 12 weeks
	Implant etonogestrel	Nexplanon	Etonogestrel	Implant (arm)	Irregular bleeding, acne, mood changes	3 years
GNRH AGONIST		Zolodex, Prostap	Goserelin, Leuprorelin	Injection	Menopause symptoms	Monthly or 3 monthly
GNRH ANTAGONIST (tablets, new)		Ryeqo, Orilissa (US)	Relugolix-estradiol-norethisterone	Tablets	Hot flushes, headaches, mood changes	Daily tablets
AROMATASE INHIBITORS		Femara	Letrozole	Oral tablets	Bone loss, joint pains, menopause symptoms	Daily

*It is important to remember that not everyone will experience all these symptoms, and not all symptoms will last for the duration of the treatments. Bleeding particularly often settles down after the first few cycles. These tablets can be helpful with a mood diary to recognize which *type* of progesterone-based medications or hormone treatments caused which particular mood symptoms.

Oestrogen-based treatments

The combined oral contraceptive pill (COCP) provides both oestrogen and progesterone to suppress the ovaries from producing oestrogen, thereby reducing overall circulating levels. This suppression halts ovulation (hence its contraceptive effect), reduces activity of oestrogen-sensitive pain receptors and slows the growth of endometrial plaques. It does not make endometriosis disappear; rather, it places the disease into a sedative state. The goal is to reduce pain and improve quality of life.

The COCP can help with menstrual pain, dyspareunia (pain during intercourse) and non-cyclical pain. It is available in many different formulations. Traditionally, it is prescribed with a seven-day break to allow a lighter withdrawal bleed (not a true period since no ovulation occurs). For women whose cyclical symptoms remain problematic, the COCP can be taken continuously to reduce or eliminate bleeding.

Evidence suggests that fertility is not affected overall once a woman stops using the COCP. A key advantage of the combined pill is that oestrogen can balance progesterone and offset some progesterone-related side effects. For this reason, the COCP is often a first-line treatment and is also useful in managing other gynaecological conditions such as dysfunctional bleeding, primary dysmenorrhoea and adenomyosis (see page 201).

Progesterone-only treatments

Progesterone treatments are used to reduce endometriosis pain by thinning the endometrial tissue and plaques. They do not eliminate the disease but place lesions into a sedative state. Sustained higher progesterone levels suppress ovulation and oestrogen production, pause the menstrual cycle and thin the uterine lining. This reduces pain and helps slow progression.

Progesterone (or synthetic progestins) are well known for side effects including weight change, acne and mood disturbance. However, there are multiple forms and doses available. Remember: an intolerance to one progestin does not mean an intolerance to all progestins.

Common delivery methods include:

- IUS (uterine system, commonly called the hormonal coil): Levonorgestrel (Mirena).
- Tablets: Medroxyprogesterone acetate (Provera, Depo-Provera), Norethisterone, Drospirenone (Yasmin), Norethindrone (Camila).
- Implant: Etonogestrel (placed in the arm).

GnRH analogues

Gonadotropin-releasing hormone (GnRH) analogues (agonists and antagonists) target the brain-ovary axis, switching off hormonal stimulation at the higher source to induce a state similar to menopause. Targeting the fuse box rather than the light switch is one way of looking at how GnRH analogues work.

These drugs temporarily lower oestrogen much more significantly than the other hormonal treatments. This can slow or halt disease progression and is often used when first line treatments fail. Because progesterone levels are also lowered, these drugs can be an option for women who cannot tolerate progestins.

Pregnancy

An important element to note here is that bizarrely, despite inducing a chemical menopause state, these drugs are not officially licensed as, or recognized as, a contraceptive. This is not often explained properly, and it is important to be aware of because with there being a risk of pregnancy, although very low, these are not safe to be on while pregnant. For this reason, use of additional contraceptive methods (be it barrier protection using condoms) is still needed.

Because of the side effects and strength of these chemical-changers, they are considered a second line treatment reserved for advanced disease. The side effects include all the usual menopausal-related symptoms: hot flushes, mood changes, weight change, night sweats, insomnia, reduced libido, vaginal dryness and joint stiffness. The sudden onset can feel like being plunged into menopause overnight, because this is essentially what has happened. There is no gradual transition of natural perimenopause to buffer the blow and so it can be quite a stark and profound change, particularly when we recognize how hormones aren't just influencing our pelvic region but our entirely mood, personality, drive and emotional wellbeing (see page 30).

A risk of being in an early menopausal state is bone density loss. Long-term use of GnRH analogues without hormone add-back therapy carries an increased risk of osteoporosis. Therefore, careful monitoring of how long the treatment is used and a conscious approach by the medical team to have an awareness of these risks is needed. For this reason, use of GnRH analogues is limited to between three- and six-month periods.

To mitigate side effects, additional hormone therapy (what doctors call add-back therapy) may be prescribed, e.g. norethisterone, oral contraceptives or bisphosphonates. While this may sound counterintuitive, the balance helps protect bones and reduce menopausal symptoms while still suppressing endometriosis.

Importantly, the menopausal state is not permanent. When these treatments stop, the induced menopause state stops and fertility returns (there is no long-term risk to fertility). For many women, the experience feels surreal: being in their twenties or thirties yet suddenly feeling like they are in a 60-year-old body, only to wake up six months later back in their younger state.

My story

It's no exaggeration to say that the year of my life when I was taking GnRH analogues felt like some bizarre body-swap movie. I was in my twenties with the sex drive and tissue plumpness of such, then plunged into menopause along with the flushes, vaginal dryness and stiff joints, before being brought back for two months of my 20-year-old self. Pregnancy then followed, with morning sickness and bloating and an entirely different physiological state. It truly felt like a hormonal whiplash and not a pleasant experience.

> This experience is common for many of the women I've spoken to who have been prescribed GnRH analogues. For some, these side effects come as quite a shock when no prior warning was given, and some had no idea they were being put into a temporary menopause. Others knew but weren't quite prepared for just how stark, and quick, the effects were. As discussed in Chapter 12, the side effects and impact of this treatment don't need to be feared or be seen as a reason to avoid considering this as a treatment option. For me, although a stark shock to the system, the welcome relief far outweighed the side effects and it felt like a physical holiday after eight years of being ground down by the pain in my ovaries and uterus.

Delivery methods

GnRH analogues are commonly given by injection every 28 days and often people will encounter one named Zoladex. The large needle can be unpleasant and must be administered by a trained professional. Some women (me included) have self-administered after training – a fact that often shocks people but demonstrates how desperate for relief many of us become.

There are lots of varying opinions on Zoladex and it doesn't suit everyone. For some, Zoladex brings the first real relief after years of pain. For me, it meant six blissful months with zero pain, despite the menopausal side effects. For others, though, the plunge into menopause can feel overwhelming and they aren't always aware they can also try additional hormone tablets to help with the side effects and so quickly reject the treatment choice outright.

Due to risks, GnRH analogues are typically reserved for refractory symptoms (stubborn symptoms which persist after first line approaches have failed) or used before/after surgery (especially to treat stage three or four endometriosis). Pre-surgery, they can shrink plaques; post-surgery, they can reduce recovery pain (if immediate fertility is not a priority).

Aromatase inhibitors

Aromatase inhibitors are not hormone therapies themselves but block enzymes that convert androgens into oestrogen in fatty tissues and other sites. We have cells that still produce smaller amounts of oestrogen throughout the body (away from the ovaries) and so for people struggling with other treatment options, these can be used to 'mop up' residual oestrogen, reducing the last fragments that could be causing symptoms.

They are usually prescribed as an add-on for refractory symptoms, often alongside GnRH analogues after surgery. Examples are anastrozole, letrozole and exemestane.

Aromatase inhibitors work by trying to deplete and lower oestrogen levels as much as possible, and like with GnRH analogues, these bring with them menopausal symptoms (see page 159). Rarely they can affect the liver and so it is important to discuss potential side effects with your doctor and know the signs to be mindful of. These are not commonly used medications, but may be prescribed by a gynaecologist alongside information about what side effects to be aware of.

Relugolix (Ryeqo)

This newer drug became a social media talking point when it was finally given approval to be used in the UK. It was hailed by some as a 'wonder drug' and dismissed by others as overhyped.

Relugolix was designed to combine the best features of existing medications into one pill:

- **Relugolix** (a GnRH analogue): to lower oestrogen and progesterone.
- **Estradiol**: to offset the low-oestrogen side effects.
- **Norethisterone**: to prevent the added oestrogen from stimulating endometriosis.

This drug aims to take the best parts of the ones currently in existence; the Relugolix is a GnRH analogue but doesn't need to be given by injection and has a stronger effect at lowering oestrogen and progesterone. To offset the hypo-oestrogenic effects of this the estradiol component is a synthetic top-up to make it more tolerable. Then to stop the estradiol triggering the endometriosis, the norethisterone is added. It was designed to pull all the best features of other treatments while also hoping to offset many unpleasant side effects.

The attraction? One tablet replaces multiple drugs, combining efficacy with side-effect management. Early studies suggest it can be effective, especially for women who are highly sensitive to hormonal changes. But as with all treatments, it is not 'one size fits all' and all women respond differently to it; while some may find significant relief, others may be disappointed.

Pregnancy

Most of the hormonal options are not suitable for women who are looking to conceive immediately. This is because they induce a temporary contraceptive state. Evidence shows that fertility is not damaged or compromised long term by taking these treatments, and the chance of pregnancy is not altered. For many, fertility returns quickly after stopping their use.

REBOUND ENDOMETRIOSIS

A phenomenon which is gaining increasing popularity in belief and misrepresentation amongst online community groups is 'rebound endometriosis'. It's important to note that this is not scientifically proven in medical literature, and I remain on the fence as to whether it will ever be.

Some women who have been on a contraceptive pill or hormone treatment for many years notice what feels like a surge of intense endometriosis activity when they stop taking the medication. The common story goes: a woman takes the pill from her teenage years into her twenties, stops and is suddenly floored by horrific bleeding and pain that's far worse than before.

Some people (not doctors or medical researchers) are beginning to describe this as 'rebound endometriosis', almost as though the disease returns worse than before when the treatment stops. Even before hearing the term I too was very much aware of the idea that endometriosis appears to become more aggressive after stopping the hormone treatments. The question is: is this a true phenomenon and is there any science behind this? I have seen women openly campaigning against the use of hormonal treatments; they propose that these hormone treatments *induce* this rebound phenomena and therefore people should avoid them to protect against this 'potential future progression'.

There is currently no data to show this actually happens (and I've looked). But this perception of a 'rebounding aggressive progression' does have several reasonable explanations.

As I've explained, hormone treatments don't erase or destroy endometriosis tissue; rather they put it into a dormant state. Imagine endometrial plaques are sponge-like cells and oestrogen is the water. Hormone treatments 'dry out' the sponge, shrinking the plaques. Once treatment stops and oestrogen returns, the sponge swells again, sometimes larger than before. This is not rebound progression, but disease reactivation. The sudden shift – from no pain and controlled pseudo-periods to fertile cycles with active lesions – feels like a shock.

It's important to note that the periods women have while on hormone treatments are not true periods. They're pseudo-periods: bleeding without ovulation, with a thinner endometrial lining and the bleed is a withdrawal bleed. Transitioning back to natural cycles can feel drastically different. Meanwhile, the endometriosis may have been quietly progressing in the background, unnoticed until the hormone treatments are stopped. So, it may very well be that the disease is more obvious and perceived as more aggressive upon stopping the treatments. It's important to know that had those treatments *not* been there, the progress could have been experienced even sooner and with more extensive organ damage.

When I hear people say that hormone treatments such as the contraceptive pill are 'masking the disease' as part of the anti-hormone argument, I sigh with frustration. What I hear is a woman who has not been adequately informed about what these treatments do – and this is not her fault. While treatments have masked the disease in the sense of sedating it, dulling pain and delaying surgery, they have also bought time and slowed progression. The alternative to these drugs would often be faster disease progression and more pain.

How endometriosis behaves in your body is already dictated by your cells, your oestrogen-driven pain receptors and your immune system. Treatment approaches are simply attempts to see what combination provides the best relief. **At present, nothing changes the ultimate trajectory of the disease, but some of the treatment options can slow things down.**

If we revisit the weeds in the garden analogy from page 82, we have established that a garden spoilt by weeds will never be weed-free. This is the truth for endometriosis. Using hormonal treatments is like putting weed membrane down; we are trying to limit the damage caused by the weeds (the disease); reduce their visibility and preserve the garden and the integrity of the other plants (our organs). We might also be trying to save space to potentially plant a rose bed (a pregnancy). There is no false illusion that the weed membrane has eradicated all traces of weeds, just like hormonal treatments are not promising to entirely stop or eradicate the endometrial plaques. If we lift the weed membrane and see a surge of more weeds than before it was put down, this is likely because beneath the membrane the weed's roots were spreading quietly, just unnoticed and slower. They are not rebounding aggressively because we introduced the membrane – just like endometriosis has not become worse *because* of the introduction of hormones. Had we not used the weed membrane, that garden would have been overrun within months potentially. The weed membrane bought time, possibly years, sometimes even a decade. This is the truth of how hormone treatments for endometriosis work.

This revelation was a game-changer for me, and I hope it offers some relief for you too. The end game of your disease is unfortunately determined by your body. If every woman with endometriosis had no intervention, not all would progress the same way. Some would advance rapidly, others slowly, some not at all. So, when a treatment fails or symptoms return, it isn't automatically the fault of your medical team or a false promise from a particular treatment. It reflects the unpredictability of the disease, and it's why it's important to tread carefully when comparing your journey with another woman's.

SURGERY

First laparoscopy

The first surgical procedure for many women with endometriosis is a laparoscopy, in which the consultant gynaecologist aims to diagnose and stage the disease. Small incisions are made to insert a light and camera to explore what is happening within the pelvis (see page 133).

Many women are disheartened to discover that this laparoscopy is purely diagnostic. Some consultants enter with the sole intention of looking and diagnosing, not treating. There are reasons for this (see page 135), however, it can feel anticlimactic to wake up, have the disease confirmed and then be told that another procedure will be needed later.

Surgery is often used alongside medical treatments in line with what research and evidence suggest is best. Since a laparoscopy is the most reliable way of establishing disease severity (in terms of spread), this first procedure is often necessary to map out the situation and plan accordingly.

Second laparoscopy

The aim of the second laparoscopy is to remove as many endometrial plaques as possible. Returning to the weeds analogy from page 165: you can de-weed your garden regularly, but unseen roots are often ready to spring back and some weeds are in hard-to-reach areas. Similarly, surgical removal does not promise a cure. What it does aim to do is remove active, obvious plaques which may improve pain and fertility.

For some, removing a large volume of disease allows hormone treatments to work more effectively. If you remove the bulk of the problem, residual tissue can then be better controlled with medication. Some women have one laparoscopy and then manage long-term with hormone treatments.

There are variations in surgical technique: *how* the surgeon removes the plaques and variations in whether to use hormone treatments before or after surgery. Surgery will usually aim to reduce visible plaques and remove them where possible. Previously the preferred techniques included ablation (burning) but as time has progressed it has allowed for more advanced techniques to develop. Ablation carries more risk of scarring and adhesions in response to the tissue damage, whereas more specialist surgeons now use excision as a preferred approach to removing the lesions. Excision is a highly specialized skill where the surgeon physically attempts to cut as much of the visible plaques away. Excision has shown more favourable outcomes but requires a skilled surgeon.

The surgeon may not always discuss what approach they are going to use, but it is okay to ask. Patients have choice within the NHS as to where they wish to be treated and those with stage three or four disease should ideally be under an endometriosis specialist centre.

Endometriomas

Endometriomas (blood-filled cysts on the ovaries) can be excised, drained or treated with CO_2 laser vaporization. Excision is often preferred because draining leaves behind the 'shell', which can refill. These procedures are particularly challenging where fertility is important. Endometriomas can engulf parts of the ovary, and the goal is to remove them while minimizing damage to remaining eggs.

Informed consent

For all surgery, including those explained in this book, you must give informed consent. This means that the team must discuss their plan of action with you, including the pros and cons, side effects and risks.

Hysterectomy

An important myth to debunk is that not every woman with endometriosis will require a hysterectomy and a hysterectomy is not a cure for endometriosis.

There was once a misguided belief that hysterectomy was the ultimate cure for endometriosis. It was seen as the 'final step': remove the reproductive organs, clear as much disease as possible and the problem should go away. No ovaries to stimulate, so surely no activity, right? But even after hysterectomy, endometriosis can and does persist, the relentless weed that it is.

A hysterectomy is major surgery and not to be taken lightly. Some assume that the only objection is that it will end their fertility, and women sometimes meet resistance by their medical team because of their age. Surgeons are not only reluctant for fear your future self might regret the decision to become infertile, but removal of these organs also induces surgical menopause (if ovaries are removed), which carries a higher risk of osteoporosis and longer-term health risks due to less oestrogen in the body, particularly at younger ages. Removal of the uterus also changes the position of remaining pelvic organs: the bladder, uterus and bowel normally support each other, so when one is removed shifts occur that can cause prolapse or adhesions (scar-like bands where tissues stick together after inflammation or bleeding).

For these reasons, hysterectomy is usually reserved for severe disease where endometriosis is causing major quality-of-life disruption or poses a risk to the bowel or bladder. Women usually need counselling because hysterectomy results in permanent infertility and, if the ovaries are removed, menopause. Younger women would then be strongly advised to start HRT (hormone replacement therapy) to protect bone health.

There are different types of hysterectomy: a total hysterectomy (removal of uterus and cervix) with or without removal of the fallopian tubes and ovaries (see page 231). For advanced disease, full removal is often preferred to reduce recurrence risk. During this procedure, the surgeon will also try to excise visible disease.

For some women, this marks the end of their journey with endometriosis. They adapt to HRT and, although in menopause earlier than expected, find their symptoms end. A small minority with advanced disease will find symptoms return, often within two years, usually at the vaginal vault (where the cervix is removed and the top of the vagina closed) or deep in the pelvis.

Not long ago, surgeons often refused further surgery for endometriosis after hysterectomy. I remember being told post-hysterectomy that medication was my only option. But surgical techniques keep advancing and, as I write, I am on the waiting list for further surgery to remove residual disease.

Pre- and post-surgery hormone treatments

As discussed on page 166, often the first surgery is a diagnostic laparoscopy where the surgeon assesses and stages the disease to make a plan for treatment. When it comes to a laparoscopy intended to *treat,* depending on the stage of disease the surgeon has different options and variable approaches to the surgical procedure.

While evidence is limited, some surgeons will recommend a GnRH analogue (see page 159) for six months *before* surgery. This induces menopause temporarily, helping inflammation settle and creating a 'tidier' surgical field.

GnRH analogues given *after* surgery may help with pain and recovery, but only for those not immediately trying to conceive.

Other surgical interventions

LUNA (laparoscopic uterosacral nerve ablation) is a surgical procedure to try to address pain by surgically interrupting the pelvic nerves and thus stopping the pain signals from firing. This can be used for other causes of dysmenorrhoea as well, though it is a high-risk procedure and so reserved for very advanced cases.

Presacral neurectomy targets the pain nerves to stop the detection of pain, but it is again very high risk and technical and not commonly offered.

CHAPTER SUMMARY

The way you experience endometriosis may change as hormone management shifts over time. For example, a contraceptive pill that worked for years may start causing side effects, be withdrawn from prescription or simply lose effectiveness as the disease grows. Or your symptoms may change. There is no set formula for treatment, but there are multiple options.

If one therapy doesn't work, another can be tried. Combining hormone therapy, pain relief and surgery at the right points can restore your quality of life. With better counselling and support, more women could achieve control earlier.

Importantly, it is reasonable to want to mute pain. This is not masking warning signs; it is a valid goal of treatment. That said, a change in type of pain or the arrival of new symptoms (e.g. bowel or bladder changes) may suggest progression. Women with advanced disease should be monitored in a specialist centre.

There is no single pathway for both doctors and patients to manage endometriosis due to the complexities of the disease process. Until the time comes where clinicians can better identify what type of endo patient you are (i.e. how much your own disease is influenced by immune system dysfunction, sensitivity to oestrogen, etc.), we remain in a situation of using a trial-and-error approach. Understanding early on what your own aims for treatment are (pain versus fertility) and having a solid understanding of what treatment is aiming to achieve (not to cure but to improve quality of life) sets you in a strong position for having a better response to treatments. Realizing that just because one hormone treatment may not have worked, others still might and having patience with the process can be a real pivotal shift that improves your disease journey.

Key takeaways

- Be clear whether your current goal is pain relief or fertility. If fertility is pressing, non-hormonal options and surgery may be preferable.
- If you want to try to get pregnant soon, sometimes a short pause in 'trying' can allow for a trial of hormonal treatments to improve the endometriosis and reduce the inflammation. Think short-term delay for potentially longer-term success.
- Remember: treatments aim to relieve pain and slow progression. There is no cure.
- Keep a diary for at least two to three months, noting symptoms of hormone tolerance rather than just pain. This can help to guide treatment decisions.

CHAPTER 8:

ENDOMETRIOSIS: FERTILITY AND PREGNANCY

MORE THAN A BIOLOGICAL PROCESS

For many women, fertility is more than the biological process – it's identity, hope and heartbreak intertwined. When you live with endometriosis, that relationship becomes even more complex. The myths, misinformation and misguided advice surrounding fertility can be just as painful as the physical symptoms themselves. But it doesn't need to be a story of despair; it can be one of knowledge, empowerment and the unwavering truth that understanding your body is the first step toward reclaiming control over it.

Fertility is an intensely emotive topic. The yearning for a child can feel primal, amplified by hormones that have often been thrown into chaos by the disease or its treatments. But there is hope. Endometriosis does not mean pregnancy will never happen, nor does it automatically mean that assisted reproductive technology (ART) is required.

Statistics vary, but research suggests that women with mild to moderate disease (stages one or two) have a reasonable chance of conceiving naturally, and some studies estimate success rates of up to 50 per cent. The odds decline for those with more advanced disease; the more extensive the endometriosis, the lower the likelihood of conceiving or sustaining a pregnancy without assistance. Even so, with the right interventions and support those odds can often be improved.

> **Myth busting**
>
> 'The best treatment for endometriosis is pregnancy' is outdated advice that needs retiring immediately.
>
> If we consider that endometriosis accounts for around half of all cases of infertility in women, telling someone who is already struggling to conceive that the treatment for the condition causing her infertility is the very thing she cannot do is absurd. It's like phoning a garage to say your car won't start and being told, 'Drive it here and we'll fix it.'
>
> I remember sitting in clinic after two or three miscarriages and being told, with clinical detachment, that the cure for my pain and endometriosis was simply to get pregnant. I stared at the consultant in disbelief before reminding him that I couldn't sustain a pregnancy – precisely because of the endometriosis. He shrugged and said, 'Go get IVF.' Because I already had one child, this meant paying out more than £10,000 ($13,500 USD).
>
> The second problem with the 'pregnancy cures endometriosis' myth is that the disease does not quietly vanish for nine months. It's unpredictable, invasive and often continues to cause pain and inflammation throughout pregnancy.

UNDERSTANDING INFERTILITY

Thankfully the days of cruelly branding a woman 'barren' if she struggles to conceive are gone. Infertility today is recognized as a spectrum of challenges and causes, and understanding which type you're facing helps determine the most appropriate approach and treatment.

Primary versus secondary infertility

Infertility is defined as the inability to conceive or sustain a pregnancy. It can be categorised as primary or secondary:

- **Primary infertility** refers to difficulty conceiving after one year of regular, unprotected vaginal sex, when no pregnancy has ever been achieved.
- **Secondary infertility** refers to difficulty achieving or sustaining a pregnancy after previously giving birth to a live baby. It also includes cases where pregnancies occur but end in miscarriage or loss.

People are often confused about what counts as actively trying to conceive. Primary infertility applies when conception has never occurred despite a year of regular intercourse without contraception.

Believe it or not, I've met individuals who didn't realize that conception requires vaginal penetration without contraception and that, biologically speaking, it's the man's orgasm that's essential for fertilization, not the woman's (though hers is certainly preferable for reasons beyond conception). Sex can mean different things to different people, and misconceptions still exist even among adults.

Someone may have one healthy child and then struggle for years to conceive again – or they may experience multiple miscarriages – and both scenarios count as secondary infertility.

Causes of infertility and miscarriage

Many women wonder how a condition that exists *outside* the uterus can interfere with what happens *inside* it. There are several mechanisms at play here:

- **Structural damage**: Adhesions and endometrial plaques can distort pelvic anatomy, preventing the uterus from expanding normally or blocking the fallopian tubes. If a fertilized egg cannot travel to the uterus it may implant in the tubes or on the ovary, causing an ectopic pregnancy (literally meaning 'in the wrong place').
- **Inflammation and immune response**: Chronic inflammation creates an inhospitable environment for a pregnancy. The immune system's antibodies, confused by disease activity, may misidentify an embryo as a threat. The body, designed to prioritize the mother's survival, may then end the pregnancy.

- **Associated autoimmune disorders**: Endometriosis increases susceptibility to autoimmune conditions such as lupus or antiphospholipid syndrome, both of which can produce antibodies that trigger miscarriage.
- **Ovarian involvement**: Endometriosis on the ovaries can impair egg quality, which in turn hinders fertilization or results in embryos that are not viable. Endometriomas (see page 134) may also physically obstruct ovulation.

MISCARRIAGE: THE UNSPOKEN STATISTIC

One in four pregnancies (25 per cent) end in a miscarriage, usually in the first trimester. This statistic is true for any woman, even without any underlying diagnosis. It's astonishingly common yet rarely discussed, and almost never mentioned in sex education classes.

Because it's statistically 'common', one or two miscarriages aren't usually classified as a fertility problem. Medical investigations typically begin only after three consecutive losses, what is medically classified as recurrent miscarriage. It's at this point that doctors start exploring underlying causes such as endometriosis, hormonal imbalance or autoimmune disease.

I conceived my first child within months of stopping the combined contraceptive pill I'd taken since my teens. At the time, I had no inkling of any underlying gynaecological disease I was harbouring. The pregnancy was uncomfortable but successful and I entered my next chapter of family planning blissfully unaware of what was coming. Then came miscarriage after miscarriage. True to textbook, it wasn't until the third loss that my GP began investigating and set me on the path to an endometriosis diagnosis.

Seeing those two faint pink lines – or that blue cross depending on your brand of pregnancy test – sparks an instant vision of the future: a baby name list, nursery colours, the anticipation of a growing bump. That's what makes miscarriage particularly cruel. Even after loss, the body continues to notice the declining, but still circulating, pregnancy hormone hCG for days or weeks. Morning sickness and tender breasts linger, cruel reminders of a pregnancy that's been lost.

Emotional support following miscarriage is, far too often, missing. Consultations usually focus on why it happened and what's next, both of which matter, but so does how you feel. Many women are desperate to move on and immediately ask, 'How soon can I try again?' The determination to keep going often sidelines emotional recovery.

I had six miscarriages and not once did a doctor, nurse or midwife offer counselling or even suggest mental-health support. As a doctor myself, I'm not phobic about clinical settings, but once I'm the patient, tears come easily. To my GPs, it was probably nothing new, but in a fertility clinic that visible distress should have raised concern.

Support after pregnancy loss

I strongly encourage every woman – and her partner – to attend at least one counselling session after a miscarriage. Sitting in a neutral space with someone trained to listen can reveal layers of grief or trauma that might otherwise stay buried. Ignoring that pain risks it resurfacing later, sometimes as postnatal depression (PND). And postnatal depression isn't something that only effects women who have given birth to a healthy baby.

Postnatal depression can affect anyone after a pregnancy, even one resulting in a miscarriage. The profound shift of hormones from a pregnancy state to a postnatal state (even after miscarriage) can trigger PND. People don't expect it after a miscarriage and so it can become insidious quickly if not recognized. Any concern over concentration, mood, anxiety, sleep disturbances or intrusive thoughts *must* be discussed with a professional. The NHS has a specific perinatal mental health team which doesn't have the lengthy waits that the standard mental health team has. Women can access this service quickly via their midwife or GP and very quickly get the right support and help needed.

There are excellent charities offering free emotional support after pregnancy loss. Even if you don't think you need help, speaking with someone experienced can offer unexpected relief and strength. Fertility is a marathon, not a sprint, and emotional recovery is every bit as important as the physical.

FERTILITY TREATMENTS

Egg freezing

Egg freezing is a deeply personal choice and one that involves cost, emotional weight and a complex set of factors. I'm often asked whether someone newly diagnosed with endometriosis, especially teenagers or women in their early twenties, should consider egg preservation. As a responsible clinician, I always return to the evidence, and the evidence tells us this: egg preservation is not routinely recommended for endometriosis.

Research has not shown egg freezing to significantly improve later pregnancy success rates. That doesn't mean it has no value; for some it offers reassurance or control, but it isn't a guaranteed safety net. It's essential to make the decision with full information, realistic expectations and proper medical advice.

Assisted reproductive technology (ART)

When we talk about ART – assisted reproductive technology – most people immediately think of IVF. But IVF, or in vitro fertilization, is just one approach within a much wider spectrum of fertility treatments. The term ART covers a range of medical interventions designed to help conception where natural fertilization is difficult or impossible. Depending on the specific barrier (for instance, blocked fallopian tubes) ART can bypass the problem entirely by placing a fertilized embryo directly into the uterus.

This is an entire field in itself and the many protocols, medications and techniques available can be overwhelming. Unfortunately, within the endometriosis community, ART is often poorly timed or poorly explained, offered too soon, too late or with misplaced expectations. As both a doctor and a patient, I've seen wildly inconsistent statistics, interpretations and advice. The truth is that research on when and how ART works best for women with endometriosis remains in flux. Data and protocols are constantly evolving.

That said, ART does have a legitimate and valuable role. It can improve fertility outcomes, but only when carefully planned in collaboration with your gynaecologist and, ideally, an endometriosis-aware fertility specialist. Your disease stage heavily influences which ART method is most appropriate and whether preliminary surgical management should come first. The overview of ART approaches discussed here is based on the current leading guidelines and research available.

For women experiencing secondary infertility, especially those who already have a child, NHS-funded ART is rarely available. Even for primary infertility, endometriosis as a cause doesn't automatically qualify for NHS funding.

Navigating the interface between private fertility clinics and NHS gynaecology teams can feel like walking a tightrope between two separate systems that barely communicate. Differences in expertise, data interpretation and preferred techniques mean there is no single 'right way' through this landscape.

Despite these frustrations, ART can offer hope. But it's not purely a physical process; it's also an emotional, psychological and often financial one. Understanding that dual impact is key before deciding how and when to proceed.

Intrauterine insemination (IUI)

IUI involves preparing sperm and placing them directly into the uterus around the time of ovulation. It's often recommended for women with early-stage endometriosis (stage one or two) when disease activity is limited.

Sometimes this is combined with ovarian stimulation medication to encourage egg release, helping to overcome minor mechanical barriers such as tubal adhesions or disrupted egg transport.

Controlled ovarian stimulation (COH)

This approach uses hormonal medications to stimulate the ovaries to produce multiple eggs per cycle. If mild endometriosis has affected egg release or quality, encouraging several eggs increases the chance that at least one will successfully reach the uterus for fertilization.

In vitro fertilization (IVF)

IVF is typically reserved for advanced endometriosis, when significant pelvic or tubal damage makes natural fertilization unlikely. The process stimulates the ovaries to produce multiple eggs, which are then retrieved and fertilized with sperm in a laboratory.

The resulting embryos are observed over several days and graded for quality. The best-graded embryo is transferred directly into the uterus, with the recipient primed using tailored hormone therapy to optimize implantation.

IVF bypasses many of the anatomical and inflammatory barriers that endometriosis creates, offering a viable route to conception when other options have failed.

My story

I was advised to pursue IVF quickly and told that it was my only hope before time ran out. I trusted that advice – as many patients do – without realizing how many vital steps had been skipped. I had advanced endometriosis but had never undergone excision surgery. No one discussed embryo freezing or managing the inflammation first.

£12,000 ($16,000 USD) later, after months of injections, scans and cautious optimism, I miscarried. I was broken – physically, financially and emotionally. Years later, when I finally found an endometriosis specialist, he confirmed what I'd already begun to suspect: my body had been in no state to nurture a pregnancy. The inflammation and scarring were too severe. The IVF was never likely to succeed; not because I failed, but because my care plan did.

I carried that anger for a long time. But anger doesn't change outcomes, knowledge does. That experience now fuels my determination to make sure other women are equipped with the information I lacked.

Had I known what I know now, I could have made informed choices (surgery first, hormonal preparation then IVF under the right specialist) and the story *might* have ended differently.

> The truth is that success in fertility treatment for endometriosis depends on collaboration, timing and tailored care. Your stage of disease will influence the type of intervention most likely to help. The cost will determine accessibility and the conversation between you and your medical team will shape everything that follows.

Surgery prior to IVF

Whether surgery should precede IVF is one of the most debated questions in fertility medicine. Some studies show that excision surgery (removing endometrial plaques and scar tissue) can improve IVF success rates by reducing inflammation, reopening blocked tubes and enhancing ovarian function.

Think of it like gardening. If you try to plant a new rose bed in a patch overrun with weeds, the seed may never take root. You might have better luck planting a more established sapling, but it still has to fight the weeds for space. Or you can clear the ground first, giving the rose a fair chance to thrive. You know the weed roots are there and will return, but that temporary clearance allows for time to allow the rose bed to take hold successfully.

That's what surgery can do: temporarily clear and calm the pelvic environment, allowing the embryo a better chance to implant and grow. Of course, endometriosis tends to regrow over time, but even a short window of improved pelvic health can make a significant difference to a woman's chance of conceiving.

Embryo freezing

The role of frozen embryo transfer (FET) often arises in discussions of IVF for advanced endometriosis. This is different from egg freezing (see page 176). Egg freezing is the harvesting of eggs – frozen to be used for a later date. Embryo freezing is when the eggs have been fertilized *in vitro* and rather than immediately transferred to the uterus, the established embryo (pregnancy in waiting) is frozen.

To explain why this might be needed we need to revisit the cause for the infertility. The process of IVF requires the ovaries to be heavily stimulated with hormones, particularly oestrogen. This is required to produce multiple eggs at once, sometimes 20 to 40 in a single cycle. This process can cause bloating, discomfort and, for those sensitive to oestrogen, a flare in endometriosis symptoms. IVF is a numbers game and after the initial excitement of starting with 30–40 eggs, the disappointing reality is that possibly only one or two viable embryos reach the finish line.

The challenge is that the same hormonal stimulation needed to collect eggs can also fuel the underlying disease. To counter this, many clinics use a 'pause protocol': after harvesting the eggs, they freeze the embryos and halt treatment for several months. During this pause, medication such as GnRH analogues (see page 159) are used to induce a temporary chemical menopause, allowing inflammation to settle and the pelvic environment to calm. This improves chances of the embryo transfer being received and welcomed by the uterus and pelvic region successfully.

For many women, this break improves the odds of successful implantation. However, emotionally the decision can be difficult. When you've already endured so much to reach this point, being told to wait feels counterintuitive, especially when every month feels precious. Yet taking that time often means giving your body the best possible chance for success. The pause isn't wasted time; it's preparation and a potential for improving those odds.

Additional protocols

Within ART, there's not just one path but a web of variables: different drugs, doses, timing schedules and 'add-ons'. These can include everything from additional hormone injections to immune infusions or even low-dose aspirin regimens. Many of these protocols are evidence based and directed by your specific underlying conditions.

This patient-centred approach may sound promising, but such a variety of options and information can be overwhelming. Many couples are presented with multiple options at once, often without clear explanations of the evidence behind each. When hope is high and information is dense, it's easy to feel lost in statistics and probabilities.

Here's my practical advice: ask questions, take time and research thoughtfully. More information isn't always better information, and more interventions don't always equal higher success. When in doubt, return to the central question: Will this specific step improve my chances based on the actual cause of my infertility? If the answer isn't supported by evidence, that uncertainty itself can be your answer. The best approach is always the one grounded in knowledge, not desperation.

OTHER FACTORS TO CONSIDER

Emotional support

Even as a medical professional, stepping into the surreal world of fertility clinics was unnerving. I've spent my career in hospitals, and I know their smells, their language, their rhythm. Yet walking into a fertility clinic not as a doctor but as a woman hoping to conceive felt entirely different.

It was clinical, sterile and somehow stripped of the intimacy that pregnancy is supposed to symbolize. You expect conception to happen through love, not under fluorescent lights surrounded by stainless steel and syringes.

The emotional weight of fertility treatment is immense. Fear, hope, grief and determination all coexist in a single appointment. The process is lengthy and invasive – a constant cycle of blood tests, scans, injections and waiting. Culturally, many couples still treat fertility treatment as a private matter, something to be endured quietly. That silence can make the experience even harder.

Treatment can stretch over six months to a year or more, which is an extraordinary length of time to carry one of life's hardest experiences without support.

It can quickly become a numbers game: 30 eggs collected, 20 fertilized, ten embryos survive day three. Four make it to the final grading. One or two are deemed viable for transfer.

I went into IVF brimming with optimism. Surely, I thought, if medicine was now in control, success was inevitable. At my first scan, I was absurdly proud of my ovaries – more than 30 follicles. The swelling and pain didn't matter; I believed we'd cracked it. But of those 30 eggs, only four became embryos and just one survived long enough for transfer. I remember calling the clinic an hour after they told me the others hadn't made it, convinced there'd been some mistake. How could 30 turn into only one?

The IVF process is not just physical and biological. The hormones you are exposed to affect everything: your mood, appetite, weight, sleep and perspective. Without emotional support, the toll can be devastating. Open communication with your partner, friends or a therapist isn't an overshare or burden, it's survival.

IVF brings enormous hope, and for many, it's success can be life changing. But it is not an easy road. And it is okay to admit that, more so it's vital to acknowledge and respond to this truth. Approaching treatment with emotional readiness, support and realism doesn't make you weaker; it makes you stronger and better prepared for whatever outcome follows.

Cost

I wish I could say that fertility support for women with endometriosis was universally available through the NHS. Sadly, it isn't. Even for those without children, endometriosis alone isn't always considered an automatic qualifying condition for NHS-funded IVF.

Eligibility depends on a postcode lottery of local criteria: disease stage, age, previous treatment and whether you already have a child. It's a maddeningly inconsistent system. The only definitive way to know whether you qualify is to speak directly with your gynaecologist.

For those pursuing treatment privately, the financial burden can be staggering. One cycle of IVF typically costs between £4,000 and £12,000 ($5,500 and $16,000 USD) and if it fails, the costs continue to rise with each attempt.

If you're considering private treatment, research is everything. Investigate each clinic's success rates, their specialists and – crucially – whether any of the clinicians have a genuine interest in endometriosis-related fertility. Just as not every gynaecologist specializes in endometriosis, not every fertility expert understands its nuances.

In private settings, you'll often encounter a menu of additional options – the so-called 'add-ons' – all promising to improve your chances. I was offered several, but when I pressed for evidence of their benefit, I discovered that most had none. Spending another £2,000 ($2,700 USD) on something unproven isn't a gamble everyone can afford.

Always feel entitled to ask questions such as:

> 'Why is this being done?'
> 'Will this change my outcome?'
> 'Is this backed by evidence?'

Transparency is a hallmark of a good clinic. The best will be open about costs and outcomes, others less so. Look for reviews, talk to other patients and, above all, trust your instincts.

Your medical team

Your gynaecologist should remain your anchor; the person who knows your full medical picture and can help you decide whether, when and where to pursue fertility treatment.

Fertility clinics are different from gynaecology clinics – their purpose is the process of fertilization ultimately. They do not have the tools and set-up to directly manage your underlying cause, rather they are there to work *alongside* your gynaecologist. This is often misunderstood and many women think that by going directly to the fertility clinic the underlying cause of fertility will automatically be addressed, which isn't the case.

There can be a temptation that while awaiting a confirmed diagnosis, without even having seen a gynaecologist, to 'skip some steps' and seek fertility advice alongside the NHS wait for your diagnostic laparoscopy. Just like with the rose bed and preparing the soil – approaching fertility support requires all the tools and information, so my advice would be to keep your gynaecologist in the loop.

CHAPTER SUMMARY

The world of medically assisted conception is anything but straightforward. It's filled with hope, heartbreak, complex science and enormous emotional weight.

It affects not just your body, but your mind, your relationships and your sense of self.

ART (assisted reproductive technology) has an important place for women with endometriosis. It can bring real opportunity. But it's not a one-size-fits-all solution and no single protocol could ever prescribe a universal answer. The key is individualized, coordinated care: a genuine partnership between you, your gynaecologist and (where appropriate) a fertility specialist.

Key takeaways

- There are multiple ways in which endometriosis can create fertility challenges, but there is hope to achieve a pregnancy through the use of surgery, medications and assisted reproductive technology (ART) such as IVF.
- The place for ART and its potential success is dependent on the stage of your underlying disease. This should require a conversation with both your gynaecologist and the fertility specialist; they are not one and the same.
- Surgery prior to IVF to improve chances of success is often reserved for more advanced disease and the best way to know what is right *for you* is to ask all the questions to your specific team who know what is happening *in your pelvis*.

CHAPTER 9:

FIBROIDS: MORE THAN JUST HEAVY PERIODS

COMMON YET MISUNDERSTOOD

When we talk about painful or heavy periods, the conversation nearly always turns to endometriosis. But sitting quietly in the shadow of that conversation is another condition that affects millions of women: fibroids.

Fibroids are incredibly common yet astonishingly misunderstood. They're benign tumours of the uterus, which sounds alarming until you realize that most women who have them will never even know they exist. For others, however, these growths can cause significant pain, heavy bleeding, anaemia, fertility challenges and a frustrating sense of being dismissed if their symptoms are minimized.

For years, fibroids were bundled into the catch-all category of period problems, reduced to a line in a textbook or an afterthought in clinical discussions. Even as a doctor, I once saw them in those simplistic terms, a bullet point under 'heavy periods'. It's only through lived experience, patient stories and evolving medical understanding that I've come to appreciate how uniquely impactful fibroids can be and how important it is to talk about them properly.

A SECONDARY CAUSE OF HEAVY BLEEDING

Fibroids – benign tumours of the uterus – can be debilitating, affecting quality of life and fertility, but the encouraging truth is that fibroids can be treated and often cured.

I can still picture my old medical school revision notes: the title 'Period Problems' scrawled in pink highlighter, arrows branching off to Painful Periods = Endometriosis and Heavy Periods = Fibroids. Somewhere above in smaller handwriting sat adenomyosis (see page 201) linking to both pain and heaviness. Looking back, I'm a little embarrassed by how simplified that diagram was. But it did capture one thing accurately: a map pointing toward possible causes of period disorders.

If we recall the primary and secondary causes of period pain or heavy bleeding (see page 67), endometriosis, adenomyosis and fibroids all fall under the secondary category. In other words, the pain and bleeding are not random; they are symptoms of an organic disease process within the reproductive organs.

FIBROIDS IN NUMBERS

Two key statistics help put fibroids into perspective:

1. Fibroids are extremely common – they present in as many as 60 to 90 per cent of women.
2. Only one in three of all women will ever experience symptoms or need medical attention for their fibroids.

So, while fibroids are widespread, most are harmless passengers. They often sit quietly, causing little or no disruption to menstrual cycles or fertility. If you happen to see that dramatic '90 per cent of women have fibroids' statistic splashed across social media, remember this: prevalence doesn't equal problem.

For those who do experience symptoms, these range from heavy bleeding and anaemia to pressure effects and, occasionally, fertility difficulties – all of which can be effectively managed with the right treatment.

This is why sound medical advice matters. Being told you have fibroids is not, by itself, a reason to panic or to assume you'll need a hysterectomy. Many fibroids require no treatment at all.

FIBROIDS: MORE THAN JUST HEAVY PERIODS

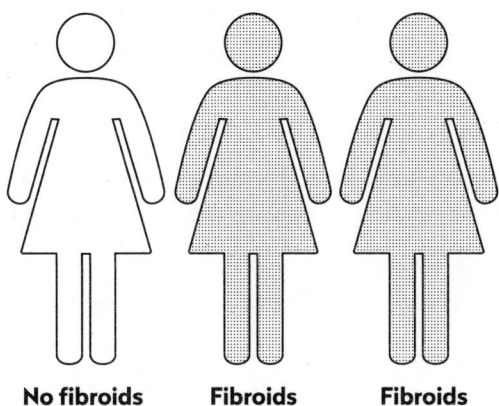

No fibroids   Fibroids   Fibroids

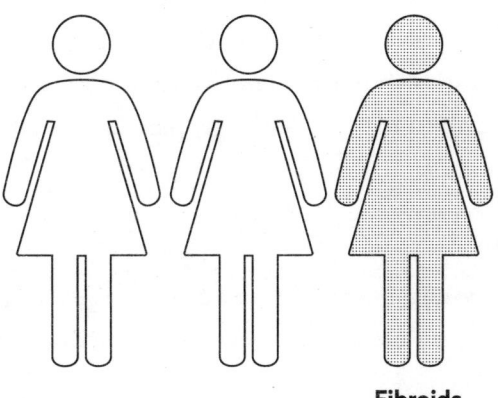

Fibroids causing problems

> **Why too many tests can cause problems**
>
> Fibroids highlight a truth about medicine that surprises many people: more scanning doesn't always mean better healthcare. Patients often ask why doctors don't simply perform full body scans each year to check for signs of disease. Besides cost, logistics and radiation risk, there's another problem: finding things that don't need fixing.
>
> The human body isn't flawless. Most of us live quite happily with benign lumps, small cysts or harmless anatomical quirks. In medicine we call these incidental findings – abnormalities that are unexpected but cause no harm.
>
> The principle 'if it isn't broken, don't fix it' applies here. Intervening where there's no problem risks creating one. Fibroids are a perfect example: common, mostly benign and best left alone unless they're actively causing trouble.

WHO GETS FIBROIDS?

Fibroids can develop in anyone with a uterus but are most common between ages 30 and 50. They tend to increase with age, particularly among women who haven't had a pregnancy.

A few key risk factors are:

- **Oestrogen exposure**: Fibroids are fuelled by oestrogen. People with higher body-fat levels have more circulating oestrogen, which can encourage fibroid growth.
- **Ethnicity**: Fibroids are significantly more prevalent among women of African-Caribbean heritage due to genetic predisposition. This same group is also more likely to experience anaemia and vitamin D deficiency, compounding the effects of heavy bleeding.
- **Genetics and environment**: Family history, hormonal fluctuations and metabolic factors all play supporting roles.

When fibroids do cause heavy bleeding, the resulting anaemia can be exhausting and lead to headaches, breathlessness, poor concentration and fainting. Severe anaemia feels as though your body is wading through quicksand, fighting harder just to function. Most cases are mild, but in high-risk groups the overlap of fibroids, anaemia and vitamin D deficiency can make symptoms far worse.

UNDERSTANDING FIBROIDS

Fibroids (also called myomas or leiomyomas) are benign tumours made up of muscle and fibrous tissue that grow in and around the uterus, particularly within its muscular layer.

Every cell in the body has a built-in regulatory system for replication. Sometimes a few cells go rogue, multiplying faster than they should but without becoming malignant. When cells maintain their original structure and behaviour, the growth is benign. When they mutate and lose control, they become malignant. Fibroids fall firmly in the benign category. They do not turn into cancer, nor do they increase the risk of uterine cancer.

Fibroids can be as small as a pea or as large as a grapefruit. Their location within the uterus determines both their name and the symptoms they cause.

Let's briefly revisit the anatomy to understand further. The uterus has a central muscle layer (the myometrium) which itself has three sub-layers:

1. **The junctional zone (JZ)**: the inner layer next to the endometrium. Its small contractions help sperm travel toward the egg, acting like a microscopic conveyor belt for conception.
2. **The middle layer**: the powerhouse of smooth muscle fibres, rich in blood vessels and nerves.
3. **The outer layer**: a thin membrane separating the uterus from the surrounding pelvic structures.

Depending on which of these layers a fibroid occupies, its impact can range from barely noticeable to severely disruptive. That's why understanding where your fibroid sits is far more meaningful than knowing how big it is.

Intramural fibroids

The most common type of fibroid, found within the middle muscle layer. Restricted in growth potential and hidden aware from the vascular endometrial tissue, they usually have few if any symptoms.

Submucosal fibroids

Situated on and near the inner layer, submucosal fibroids are close to the endometrial lining, often invading the JZ (see above). Their proximity to the endometrial lining means they disrupt the function of the endometrium, causing irregular and heavy bleeding. Submucosal fibroids can also be pedunculated and sit within the uterine space known as 'intracavity fibroids'.

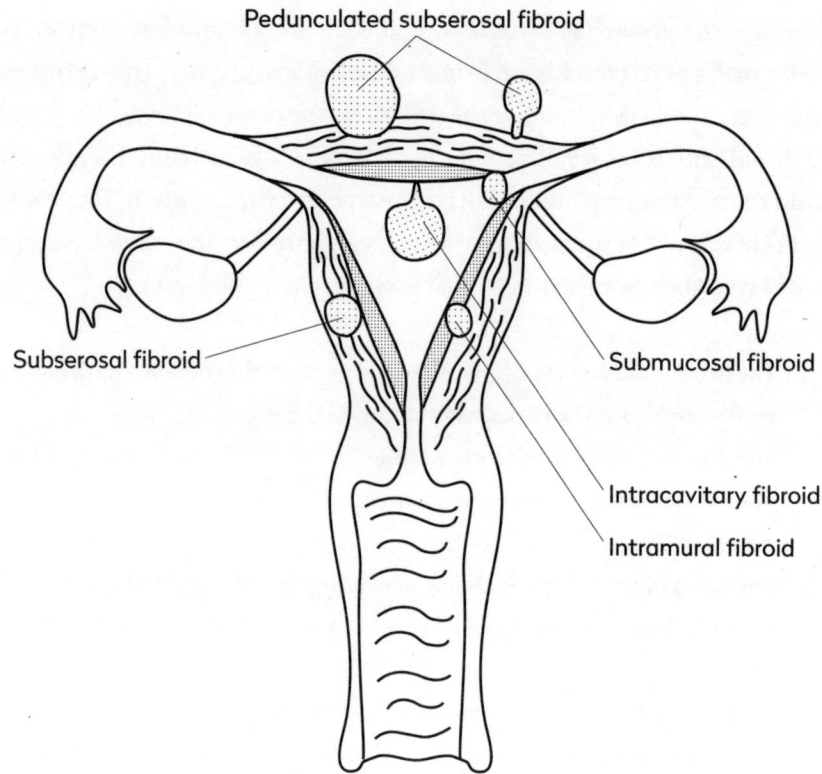

Subserosal fibroids

These are found on the outer part of the uterus, where they tend to grow quite large in the open space, as nothing is limiting them from invading it. Their growth and size encroach on the bladder and bowel and tend to cause bulk-related symptoms (see page 192).

The submucosal and subserosal fibroids can grow within the muscular layer itself or branch from a stalk of tissue, when they become known as pedunculated.

SYMPTOMS

Understanding the type and location of fibroids helps explain why they affect women so differently. Some fibroids cause no problems at all; in fact, many are discovered by accident – what doctors call an incidental finding – while scanning for something else entirely. If the fibroids aren't causing symptoms or posing risk, doctors tend to leave them alone.

When symptoms do appear, they usually fall into two categories: bleeding-related and bulk-related.

Bleeding-related symptoms

The most troublesome fibroids for bleeding are the submucosal ones, that is those sitting just beneath the inner lining of the uterus. Because they invade the endometrium and junctional zone, they disrupt the normal shedding process of menstruation. This leads to:

- Heavy or prolonged periods.
- Irregular bleeding between cycles.
- Spotting or persistent bleeding.
- Anaemia-related symptoms (fatigue, dizziness, breathlessness, headaches).

Over time, persistent heavy bleeding can deplete iron levels, leaving the body struggling to function at its usual pace. It's not 'just a heavy period'; it's a genuine medical condition that can significantly impact daily life.

Bulk-related symptoms

The bulk-related problems come from fibroids that physically enlarge the uterus or press on nearby organs. These are usually the subserosal fibroids (situated on the outer part of the uterus). Imagine filling a balloon with marbles and tennis balls – eventually it stretches, bulges and presses on whatever surrounds it. That's what fibroids can do inside the pelvis.

Depending on where they grow, fibroids may cause:

- Pressure on the bladder, leading to frequent urination or urgency.
- Pressure on the bowel, causing bloating, cramps or constipation.
- Lower back or pelvic pain.
- Visible abdominal distension.

At their most severe, fibroids can cause the uterus to enlarge so much that it resembles a pregnancy of 12 to 20 weeks. This physical expansion causing pressure symptoms on neighbouring organs is what clinicians describe as bulk symptoms.

Fertility, pregnancy and miscarriage

Fibroids can *sometimes* interfere with fertility, though this is not inevitable and, crucially, often reversible. The mechanisms that can cause problems with fertility are often due to:

- **Implantation disruption**: Fibroids that distort the uterine cavity can make it difficult for an embryo to implant or grow.
- **Sperm transport issues**: Submucosal fibroids can disrupt the junctional zone, impairing the subtle contractions that help guide sperm toward the egg.
- **Tubal obstruction**: A fibroid near the fallopian tube opening can physically block the egg or sperm from reaching each other.
- **Immune response**: The body may interpret fibroid tissue as foreign, triggering inflammation that can interfere with implantation or increase miscarriage risk.

But – and this is vital – these barriers are not absolute. The presence of fibroids does not mean a woman can't become pregnant or can't have a healthy uncomplicated pregnancy or labour. With the right treatment, many women conceive naturally once fibroids are removed or reduced. Assisted-reproduction methods such as IVF can help when physical obstruction remains or when time is a factor, but for many, fertility returns once the uterine environment is restored.

That said, the presence of fibroids can make the uterus a little more temperamental when pregnant. Because these growths occupy the muscular layer, they can increase uterine irritability, leading to cramping, more noticeable Braxton Hicks contractions or – rarely – labour that doesn't progress as expected. Occasionally, a caesarean section is required if the uterus struggles to contract effectively.

Always tell your obstetric team if you have, or have had, fibroids. It helps them anticipate potential complications during labour or delivery.

During both of my successful pregnancies, I experienced what was later called an irritable uterus. From around 20 weeks onwards, I had intense, painful contractions that mimicked early labour. I was constantly reassured that everything was fine, but the lack of explanation left me feeling unseen and dismissed. Only years later did I discover, buried in my medical notes, that I'd had a significant fibroid irritating my uterine wall the entire time.

Size versus location – does size matter?

In the case of fibroids, it's not about size or number, it's all about location. A single small fibroid in the wrong place can cause more disruption than ten large ones tucked harmlessly into the uterine wall. One pea-sized submucosal fibroid can trigger heavy bleeding or infertility, while someone else's grapefruit-sized intramural fibroid may cause no symptoms at all.

What truly matters is how the fibroids are affecting you – the bleeding, the pain, the impact on quality of life. That's what guides treatment decisions, not the numbers on a scan.

GETTING DIAGNOSED

Fibroids can be diagnosed in several ways, and the path to that diagnosis often depends on how you present to your GP or gynaecologist.

The incidental discovery

Many fibroids are found by chance during scans for other reasons, such as fertility assessments, pregnancy ultrasounds or investigations for unrelated pelvic pain.

GP assessment

If you visit your GP with heavy, irregular or painful bleeding, they'll first determine whether the problem is primary (underlying disease) or secondary (caused by a condition such as fibroids, endometriosis or adenomyosis). The GP will look for clues leading them to a potential secondary underlying cause.

Your doctor may ask about:

- Cycle length and regularity.
- Period flow intensity and duration.
- Intermenstrual bleeding (bleeding between periods).
- Pain, cramping and fatigue.
- PMS symptoms or hormonal fluctuations.
- Current contraception or hormone therapy.
- Family history, including ethnic background.

Keeping a period diary for at least six months is invaluable. Record days of bleeding, heaviness, pain and mood changes throughout each month. These notes can provide diagnostic clues and inform future treatment choices.

While less relevant for the purpose of diagnosis, I always say if keeping a period symptom diary then include PMS symptoms and whether you are on any hormonal contraceptives. This can be invaluable when considering future treatment options. Recognizing if you are more sensitive to oestrogen or progesterone surges can really help you make informed choices about hormone treatments should you need to later down the line.

Physical examination

Your GP may examine your abdomen and perform a bimanual examination – pressing one hand on the abdomen while inserting two fingers into the vagina to feel the uterus. This helps identify whether the uterus feels enlarged, firm or irregular.

In clinical shorthand, we sometimes describe the uterus's size in pregnancy weeks. For example, a uterus enlarged by fibroids might be recorded as 'equivalent to 14 weeks pregnant'. It's simply a medical reference to indicate size, not a comment on actual pregnancy status.

Imaging and tests

The first-line investigation is usually an ultrasound scan because it is relatively quick, low risk and good at identifying the fibroids. This can be done one of two ways:

- Transabdominal (over the tummy)
- Transvaginal (a probe inserted into the vagina for a closer view)

These scans reveal the size, number and location of fibroids.

In some cases, your GP may arrange a hysteroscopy (using a small camera through the cervix) for a direct look inside the uterus. A laparoscopy (keyhole surgery) is rarely needed for diagnosis alone and is generally reserved for treatment or complex cases.

If anaemia is suspected, a simple blood test can check iron and haemoglobin levels to assess how much the fibroids are affecting your overall health.

MANAGEMENT OPTIONS

Many women with fibroids will have no symptoms and not need intervention; not all fibroids need removing.

Any interventions, particularly surgical, carry risk and disturbing the uterine tissues can sometimes make problems worse or cause secondary problems, so your doctor will advise on the best course of action based on your symptoms. If your fibroids do need treatment, there are multiple options available and fibroids can be cured.

If you are facing treatment for fibroids, a useful first question is: What is my priority right now: fertility or symptom control (bleeding/pain)? Because many treatments work by adjusting hormones, your goals and timelines (e.g. planning pregnancy soon vs later) will shape the plan.

Even if your overall priority is fertility, it's worth considering whether you're willing to wait six months to a year before 'trying' to address the fibroids and improve your chances of pregnancy. As frustrating as it can be, sometimes taking a few months out from 'trying' allows the team to improve the uterine conditions to optimize the chances of successful implantation.

Non-hormonal medications

There are some very effective types of medications that work very well at targeting the pain and bleeding associated with fibroids, without affecting fertility:

- **Tranexamic acid**: helps blood to clot more effectively, reducing heavy menstrual loss and the risk of anaemia. Side-effects are usually mild (e.g. nausea, tummy upset).
- **Mefenamic acid** (an NSAID/non-steroidal anti-inflammatory): lowers prostaglandins to reduce pain and menstrual flow. Can irritate the stomach; take with food and follow prescribing advice.

Hormonal medications

These aim to temper oestrogen's effect on the uterus, shrinking fibroids and easing bleeding. These are often contraceptive by their nature but can help provide a break to allow blood levels to restore and the fibroids to shrink, which can provide some mental relief as well as a physical break from the symptoms.

- **Combined oral contraceptive pill** (oestrogen + progestogen): often reduces flow and period pain.
- **Oral progestogen**: thins the endometrial lining to curb heavy bleeding.
- **Injected progestogen** (e.g. three-monthly depot): can suppress bleeding. May cause irregular spotting or amenorrhoea, weight change and mood effects. Fertility may take time to return once stopped.
- **GnRH analogues** (e.g. goserelin): induce a temporary chemical menopause to shrink fibroids and calm bleeding, often used as a pre-surgery bridge. Not a contraceptive; additional contraception is required. Menopausal-type side effects are common while on treatment.

There is also a medication called Esmya (ulipristal acetate) which is reserved for very severe fibroids in women who are not menopausal but can't have surgery. It's used to try to shrink the fibroids but there is a high risk of liver damage and so it is used as a 'last reserve' or where surgical approaches aren't appropriate. Regular monitoring with blood tests to observe the liver is needed while on this treatment.

Fibroid removal

Intervention to remove a fibroid physically can be done via surgery or non-surgical procedures. Any physical intervention carries risks of scarring and damaging the underlying uterine tissue, which is why these are not first-line options but are reserved for more severe cases. The preservation of fertility as an importance to the patient is very much considered when considering these options.

Surgical options

- **Myomectomy**: surgical removal of fibroids while preserving the uterus.
    - Approach: often laparoscopic (keyhole), sometimes open surgery depending on size/location.
    - Pros: targets the problem; preserves fertility potential.
    - Cons: bleeding/cramping post-op; recurrence is possible. Not every fibroid is reachable/suitable.

- **Hysteroscopic resection**: instruments passed through the cervix to shave submucosal fibroids inside the uterine cavity.
    - Pros: no abdominal incisions; day-case; fertility-sparing.
    - Cons: best for submucosal lesions; may require repeat passes.
- **Hysteroscopic morcellation**: specialist technique that removes intracavitary fibroid tissue in one pass.
    - Pros: potentially faster than other options with less risk of trauma to surrounding tissue.
    - Cons: availability depends on local expertise.

Non-surgical interventions

- **Uterine artery embolization (UAE)**: interventional radiology procedure that blocks the fibroid's blood supply, starving it of oxygen so it shrinks.
    - Pros: no uterine incisions; effective for larger or fewer dominant fibroids; usually short hospital stay.
    - Cons: cramping post-procedure; fertility impact remains an area of evolving evidence – discuss if pregnancy is a goal.
- **Endometrial ablation**: destroys the uterine lining (via heat/laser/balloon) to reduce heavy bleeding.
    - Pros: quick procedure, often day-case; effective for bleeding control.
    - Cons: not suitable if future pregnancy is desired; can increase miscarriage/implantation risks later.

Emerging techniques

Most women will find relief or support with the above-mentioned approaches. However, there are other highly specialized options available in select centres (with limited long-term fertility data). These include MRI-guided percutaneous laser ablation and ultrasound-guided radiofrequency ablation. If you're considering these, ask specifically about evidence, outcomes and fertility impact.

Hysterectomy and menopause

Some women will have a successful myomectomy and their fibroids won't return. However, if fibroids do return and if pregnancy is not a goal, or if symptoms remain severe despite other treatments, hysterectomy can be a definitive cure by removing the organ that hosts the fibroids. This can be an immediate relief and an absolute release for some women. Gynaecologists will need to discuss and explore leaving the ovaries to protect women from premature menopause (see Chapter 12). A total hysterectomy removing all the gynaecological organs would often require the additional use of HRT to protect women from the complications of early menopause: osteoporosis, cardiovascular disease risk and symptoms of menopause.

It's worth noting that fibroids often shrink by themselves with the onset of menopause (as oestrogen levels dwindle with the transition into menopause, so do the fibroids).

CHAPTER SUMMARY

Living with any condition that is linked to hormones and is compounded each month with heavy bleeding and poses a risk to fertility can feel overwhelming and daunting. But fibroids can be cured, managed and overcome. Most women never experience serious symptoms, and for those who do, effective treatments exist – from simple medication to minimally invasive procedures. Fibroids are benign; they don't increase cancer risk, and with menopause they often shrink naturally.

For those navigating infertility, hope is very real. With coordinated care and accurate information, many women achieve the family and quality of life they once thought impossible.

Key takeaways

- Fibroids are benign growths within the uterus and can affect up to 90 per cent of women; however *problematic fibroids* (those causing symptoms needing medical support) only affect 30 per cent of all women.

- Many women with fibroids can achieve a natural, successful pregnancy.
- There are multiple options for treating fibroids and they can be cured. Medications, surgery and interventional procedures are available to help improve symptoms, enhance quality of life and even cure fibroids.

CHAPTER 10:
ADENOMYOSIS: NOT JUST THE THIRD WHEEL

WHAT IS ADENOMYOSIS?

If endometriosis and fibroids are the headline acts of menstrual disruption, then adenomyosis is the backing singer. Adenomyosis is just as troublesome and just as capable of hijacking a woman's quality of life as its better-known counterparts, but it often goes unrecognized. This underdiagnosed and often misunderstood condition is something of a third wheel in headlines to endometriosis and fibroids but remains stubbornly its own entity.

While endometriosis involves tissue similar to the endometrium growing outside the uterus, and fibroids are fibrous tumours within the uterine muscle, adenomyosis occurs when endometrial-like tissue grows within the uterine muscle itself (the myometrium). It's often simplified as 'endometriosis within the muscle wall'. This misplaced tissue causes inflammation, swelling and cyclical bleeding within the muscular wall, which in turn disrupts the uterus's ability to contract, sustain pregnancy and maintain structure. The result? Painful, heavy periods, fertility problems and a uterus that feels less like a strong, coordinated organ and more like a bruised, exhausted muscle.

Who it affects

Adenomyosis affects around 10–20 per cent of women (roughly one in five) and accounts for a similar proportion of infertility cases. There is significant overlap with endometriosis and many women have both conditions simultaneously. The same cellular dysfunction that triggers one can often spark the other.

Just like endometriosis, adenomyosis can be silent. Some women live symptom-free or attribute their heavy or painful periods to being simply 'normal for them'. Of course, not every woman with adenomyosis needs to know she has it. If the condition isn't disrupting her quality of life, fertility or physical wellbeing, then intervention may not be necessary. However, for many women, the problems extend far beyond 'just heavy periods'. Fertility struggles, recurrent miscarriages and difficulties in pregnancy can be the first clues that adenomyosis is silently at play.

SIGNS AND SYMPTOMS

Adenomyosis is the presence of endometrial-like tissue inside the muscular wall of the uterus, which fundamentally alters its architecture. The once smooth, strong myometrium becomes inflamed and irregular, its ability to contract properly during menstruation or labour compromised.

This structural disruption affects women in the following ways:

- Periods become heavier and more painful due to internal bleeding and inflammation.
- Implantation of embryos becomes more difficult as the uterine environment is less stable.
- Pregnancy may be at higher risk of miscarriage, particularly in early stages.

The junctional zone – the delicate interface between the endometrium and myometrium (see page 189) – is also affected. Normally this zone helps sperm move toward the egg through gentle rhythmic contractions. When adenomyosis distorts this layer, conception itself can be hindered simply by failure to deliver the sperm to the waiting egg.

Adenomyoma versus adenomyosis

The presence of the ectopic endometrial-like tissue can take on two distinct patterns: focally placed or diffusely scattered:

- **Focally placed**: a single lump known as an adenomyoma.
- **Diffusely scattered**: spread throughout the muscle wall and known as adenomyosis.

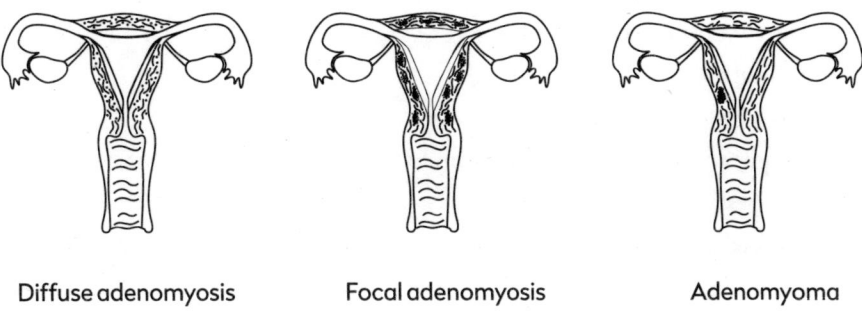

Diffuse adenomyosis   Focal adenomyosis   Adenomyoma

This distinction matters because it influences management options. An adenomyoma behaves more like a fibroid and may be removed surgically, whereas diffuse adenomyosis embedded throughout the uterine wall is more complex to treat and less amenable to surgical intervention.

The key difference between an adenomyoma and a fibroid lies in cell type and behaviour. Fibroids are made of smooth muscle and fibrous tissue that don't shed or bleed; adenomyomas contain endometrial-like tissue that responds to the hormones and so do shed and bleed. Every month, this ectopic tissue tries to respond to hormonal signals, leading to swelling, breakdown and inflammation – a small internal storm that repeats cycle after cycle.

As with endometriosis, this chronic inflammation can trigger our immune responses, leading to scarring that can disrupt fertility and increase miscarriage risk. The uterine muscle – a structure designed for strength, elasticity and precision – becomes tender, boggy and fatigued.

Symptoms

At its mildest, adenomyosis may cause no symptoms at all or only slightly heavier periods. At its worst, it can lead to debilitating pain, profound fatigue and recurrent pregnancy loss.

Common symptoms include:

- Heavy or prolonged bleeding.
- Painful periods (dysmenorrhoea).
- Pelvic bloating or pressure.
- Fatigue and anaemia-related symptoms (breathlessness, headaches, dizziness).
- Miscarriage or infertility.

The uterus itself may feel enlarged but soft ('boggy') in contrast to the hard, bulky texture typical of fibroids.

Like with endometriosis, any process that is triggering an inflammatory response has subtle ripples throughout the body: aches, fatigue, joint pains, headaches. These symptoms may be less obviously related to the pelvis but are still impactful.

GETTING DIAGNOSED

Adenomyosis is often discovered while investigating fertility challenges or recurrent miscarriages. It should be one of the key diagnoses on a GP's radar when assessing a woman presenting with painful or heavy periods, especially those over 30. This is because the prolonged exposure to oestrogen with age increases the development of adenomyosis, along with childbirth (pregnancy changing the lining of the uterine layers).

During a clinical exam, a GP or gynaecologist may feel that the uterus is enlarged and boggy, i.e. it feels soft, sponge-like and tender, rather than the firm, muscular texture associated with fibroids. A healthy uterus without problems should be difficult to feel at all because it's usually small and hidden, protected by the pubic bone. Pregnancy, fibroids and adenomyosis can increase the size and texture of a uterus as follows, which is a useful guide for doctors conducting an examination:

- Enlarged but smooth – suspect pregnancy.
- Enlarged, firm and bulky – suspect fibroids.
- Enlarged but boggy – suspect adenomyosis.

The next step is usually an ultrasound, most often a transvaginal ultrasound scan (see page 132) that provides a clearer image of the uterine wall and its structure. This can suggest changes consistent with adenomyosis. In some cases, an MRI interpreted by a specialist can confirm the suspicion with greater detail, showing irregular thickening within the uterine muscle.

Unlike fibroids or endometriosis, adenomyosis can't easily be visualized with a laparoscopy (see page 133). The disease lives within the muscle wall – not on the outer surface – so there's little to see from the outside. Only after a hysterectomy, when the uterus is examined under a microscope, can the diagnosis be confirmed with certainty.

For most women, however, the combination of symptoms, imaging and examination findings provides enough evidence to guide treatment.

MANAGEMENT OPTIONS

Adenomyosis is a hormone-driven intruder fuelled primarily by oestrogen, so the management plan for adenomyosis usually involves controlling hormones, easing symptoms and preserving fertility where possible.

Many women with adenomyosis are in their thirties or forties and at a stage where fertility decisions become particularly significant. The question often becomes: Do I want to manage the symptoms, protect fertility or both – and for how long?

Treatment approaches generally fall into three categories:

- Non-hormonal medication
- Hormonal therapy
- Surgical or procedural options

Non-hormonal medications

The following focus on symptom control, particularly heavy bleeding and pain:

- **Tranexamic acid**: supports blood clotting, helping to lighten heavy flow and reduce anaemia.
- **NSAIDs (non-steroidal anti-inflammatories)** such as ibuprofen or mefenamic acid: lower prostaglandin levels, easing both cramping and bleeding. Best taken with food to protect the stomach; not suitable in pregnancy or suspected pregnancy.

Hormonal medications

Hormonal therapies aim to suppress oestrogen (the disease's main fuel) and boost progesterone's shrinking effect on the endometrial tissue. These approaches can slow progression, shrink affected tissue and reduce pain and bleeding. They aim to create a sedative state to buy time, ease symptoms and help with fertility planning, rather than to cure. The options are:

- **IUS** (uterine system, commonly called the hormonal coil) delivers slow-release progestogen and can help thin the endometrial lining, making periods lighter. This works really well for some women but can cause erratic periods or stop periods altogether. It is a contraceptive device so is reserved for women not currently wanting to conceive. The strong influx of progesterone in its synthetic form brings a wave of side effects which some women really struggle with; these include weight gain, mood changes and erratic bleeding.
- **Combined oral contraceptives** deliver both oestrogen and progesterone to act as a contraceptive, suppressing ovulation, reducing the endometrial lining and hopefully targeting the pain and heavy periods.
- **GnRH analogues** are the chemical-menopause-inducing drugs. These injections suppress oestrogen significantly, causing an artificial menopausal

state (which is reversible) in an attempt to shrink the disease and shut it down while on the treatment. As with any of the treatments, this doesn't guarantee the disease won't continue to grow (it can and often does return after stopping these drugs). However, the temporary relief from the excessive bleeding and pain can be helpful and is also used a lot in fertility plans (see page 171). GnRH can also be used prior to surgery to help reduce the disease, which helps prepare the body to improve outcomes. GnRH analogues don't have a long-term impact on fertility and, even though this treatment induces a chemical menopause, it's not technically classed as a contraceptive, so additional contraception methods are still needed.

Surgical and procedural approaches

Surgery has a more limited role in adenomyosis than in fibroids or endometriosis because the disease is embedded within the muscle wall. To begin trying to dissect out the affected tissue carries great risk of bleeding and irreparable damage to the uterus. That said, certain procedures do have a role depending on severity and goals:

- **Adenomyomectomy**: the removal of a localized adenomyoma (a single lump) while preserving the rest of the uterus. This can improve fertility and relieve symptoms but isn't suitable for diffuse adenomyosis, which would require extensive excision.
- **Endometrial ablation:** uses heat, laser or hot-water balloons to destroy the inner uterine lining, reducing heavy bleeding. This is effective for symptom control but not appropriate for women who wish to conceive as it increases miscarriage risk and can worsen pain in some cases.
- **Hysterectomy**: removing the uterus eliminates the disease completely, offering permanent relief from pain and bleeding. However, it also ends fertility and induces surgical menopause, bringing associated risks and side effects (see page 227).

For women with both endometriosis and adenomyosis, hysterectomy can resolve the adenomyosis component but not necessarily prevent endometriosis recurrence elsewhere. Thorough discussion and shared decision-making are key.

FERTILITY

Adenomyosis can make conception and pregnancy more challenging by disrupting uterine contractions, altering the uterine lining and increasing miscarriage risk. But these challenges are not absolute barriers – with the right approach, many women go on to conceive and deliver healthy babies.

Assisted reproductive techniques (ART)

There is an adapted role for IVF with adenomyosis. Assisted reproductive techniques (ART) can attempt to achieve a pregnancy, and there are different approaches available depending on the underlying cause of infertility. For example, intrauterine insemination (IUI) is an artificial method of helping the sperm meet the egg within the uterus, to help where there is a barrier of some sort stopping this from happening. The sperm and egg fertilize within the uterus itself, whereas in vitro fertilization (IVF) takes the sperm and egg, fertilizes them in the lab and then transfers a ready-formed embryo into the uterus. There are multiple other ways of carrying out these processes, and protocols to adapt the process in response to each couple's individual medical circumstances.

In order to retrieve eggs to be fertilized in IVF, the woman is injected with a very large volume of oestrogen to prime and stimulate many ovarian follicles to release multiple eggs. It is not uncommon to stimulate 30–40 eggs, but it may be that only three or four end up being fertilized, and from there only one (if any) embryos are suitable for transfer. With these odds in mind, it can be a very intense emotional journey as well as a physically demanding one.

Because this process requires large volumes of oestrogen to stimulate the eggs, this seems counterintuitive: pumping a woman full of the hormone that causes the disease in the first place. One way the process of IVF is adapted for women with adenomyosis is to take a pause after the oestrogen-surges, rather than immediately proceeding to transfer an embryo into what is likely now an even more inhospitable environment littered with inflammation and ectopic endometrial cells. The embryos are frozen ready for transfer at a later date and the woman is put onto GnRH analogues to induce a chemical menopause to allow the uterine conditions to calm, reset and settle the inflammation inevitably happening in response to the oestrogen.

Trying to explain this pause to someone who is desperately trying for a baby (especially telling them that they may have to go into a temporary menopausal state) can sometimes not land well – particularly if the reasons for this are not communicated clearly. If you are going through this process, understanding why certain options have been taken is key and gives you the tools to ask questions and gain more clarity. (For further information, turn to Chapter 8 on pages 171–84.)

PREGNANCY

During pregnancy, adenomyosis can contribute to an irritable uterus, leading to early contractions, discomfort or slower labour progression. The condition may slightly increase the risk of miscarriage (particularly before 20 weeks) and the likelihood of needing a caesarean section.

The uterus's ability to expand and contract efficiently is sometimes compromised by the disease's scarring and inflammation. Many women, however, experience completely normal pregnancies, particularly when the condition is mild or well managed beforehand. As with any health condition, you should always make your midwife and team aware in the early consultations. Your obstetric team need to know all your medical history and this includes things like adenomyosis, endometriosis and fibroids. Share as much information as you can (although they should have access to your notes). They can then decide whether this needs to be monitored and considered as your pregnancy progresses and inform decisions about vaginal delivery versus caesarean section.

CHAPTER SUMMARY

Adenomyosis is a significant cause of painful, heavy periods and fertility struggles, but it's not without solutions. For some, symptom management brings lasting relief; for others, a hysterectomy represents the long-awaited end to years of pain and disruption.

While there's currently no complete cure short of surgery, the combination of modern fertility techniques, hormonal therapies and minimally invasive procedures has given women more options – and more hope – than ever before.

With compassionate care, informed choice, and a willingness to challenge 'normalized' suffering, it's entirely possible for women with adenomyosis to reclaim control of their bodies, their fertility and their futures.

Key takeaways

- Adenomyosis has an overlap in symptoms and similar impact to endometriosis and it is often described as 'endometriosis within the uterus muscle layer', causing pain, infertility and impact on quality of life.
- Advancing techniques to manage the disease mean there is hope for fertility and improving symptoms, with a hysterectomy offering the only definitive cure.
- Women with adenomyosis often have an overlap of endometriosis and so treatments and support need to recognize the entire disease activities happening, with treatments being predominantly hormone-based.

CHAPTER 11:
POLYCYSTIC OVARY SYNDROME AND PRIMARY OVARIAN INSUFFICIENCY

Polycystic ovary syndrome (PCOS) and primary ovarian insufficiency (POI) are often misunderstood and frequently under-discussed, yet deeply impactful on women's health, fertility and quality of life. These conditions may not cause the same level of physical organ damage as endometriosis, adenomyosis or fibroids but they can profoundly affect mental health, identity and the sense of control over one's own body.

POLYCYSTIC OVARY SYNDROME (PCOS)

Let's start by myth busting PCOS: having cysts on your ovaries does not mean you have polycystic ovary syndrome. The key word here is 'syndrome'.

PCOS is a combination of polycystic ovaries along with other symptoms as part of a syndrome that is due to the additional presence of higher than usual androgen hormones (male hormones). Many women have multiple cysts and even varying cycles where sometimes multiple follicles mature, releasing multiple eggs (which can result in conceiving non-identical twins). The presence of multiple cysts does not determine a diagnosis of PCOS.

The classic diagnostic criteria require at least two of the following to be present:

- Polycystic ovaries (multiple small follicles visible on ultrasound)
- High androgen (male hormone) levels, either through blood tests or physical signs such as facial hair, acne or hair thinning
- Irregular or absent periods

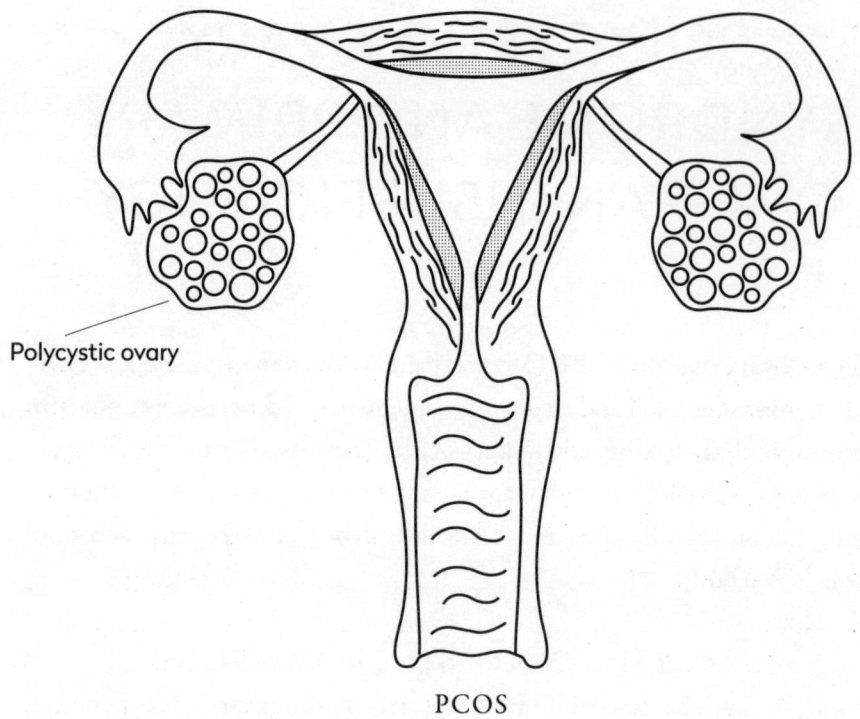

PCOS

I learned this lesson personally – and rather dramatically – in my early twenties. While a medical student, I was admitted to hospital with severe pelvic pain, thought to be appendicitis or ovarian torsion. It turned out to be a ruptured ovarian cyst (ovarian cysts commonly rupture; small ones can rupture without women even noticing, larger ones can cause immense pain and don't usually require treatment except pain relief to help until the fluid has been re-absorbed by the body). A ruptured cyst isn't life-threatening, but can be very painful. However, the symptoms early on can mimic an ectopic pregnancy or ovarian torsion, both of which *can be* a medical emergency. Therefore, any significant pain, even for those who are used to cysts rupturing, should always lead to getting the ovaries checked.

When this happened to me, the pain was excruciating, like being burned from the inside out. During the investigations, a junior doctor glanced at my scan, saw multiple cysts and casually told me – in a corridor, no less – that I had PCOS. No explanation. No plan. Just instant panic and fear from me. It wasn't until a follow-up appointment with a sensible GP that I learned the truth: I had polycystic ovaries, but not polycystic ovary syndrome. My hormone levels were normal, my cycles were regular and I had none of the other hallmarks. The irony being I was incorrectly diagnosed with one period disorder while I genuinely did have another one is not lost on me!

The reality of PCOS

PCOS affects around one in ten women, yet more than half may not realize they have it until they struggle to conceive. For some, the symptoms are subtle; for others, they're life-altering: irregular periods, unwanted hair growth, acne, weight gain or infertility.

PCOS is a whole-body condition, not just a reproductive one. The hormone imbalances – particularly raised testosterone and insulin – can ripple across every system, influencing mood and metabolism, as well as leading to long-term health risks.

The condition often leads to:

- Irregular or absent ovulation (and therefore fewer periods)
- Hirsutism (increased hair on the face, chest or back)
- Weight changes
- Oily skin or acne
- Fertility challenges

The higher androgens (male hormones) can be far more problematic for women than the periods themselves and cause excessive weight gain, facial hair, acne and coarse features. For teenage girls and young women this can have a profound impact on mental wellbeing, particularly if they don't recognize this is due to an underlying health condition.

PCOS can affect fertility, although the chances for success with the right treatment are favourable. However, many women don't even realize they have

PCOS until they have difficulty conceiving and the investigations into this identify PCOS. For some women, this is the lightbulb moment; the penny drops and they look back, recognizing years of challenges with their weight, feeling uncomfortable because of facial hair and erratic periods – it all suddenly makes sense.

Living with PCOS

PCOS is a full-body disease that extends beyond the irregular periods, fertility and hirsutism features. It's also different from the other disorders that cause pain and heavy bleeding; the erratic periods and systemic features are due to multiple hormone imbalances causing havoc not just in the short term but increasing longer-term health risks as well.

Periods can become irregular or even absent altogether and are often anovulatory, meaning ovulation hasn't occurred (i.e. no egg is released). The hormone imbalances see higher insulin, higher testosterone, higher levels of LH and even higher levels of prolactin.

High levels of insulin and testosterone disrupt the delicate hormone cycle that coordinates ovulation. The result is irregular or absent periods and an increased risk of longer-term complications such as:

- Type 2 diabetes
- Cardiovascular disease
- Endometrial (uterine) cancer

Hormones don't just influence the target organs; they have widespread effects on our mental wellbeing, drive, interests, libido and energy. PCOS can profoundly influence and alter who women are in many senses.

Irregular periods can also lead to an increased risk of endometrial cancer. This is because for women who have fewer than three or four periods a year their endometrial tissue isn't 'turning over' the way it should, which is associated with a higher lifetime risk of endometrial cancer. Our cells like to regenerate and turn over. Anything that disrupts this 'status quo' can potentially have a consequence somewhere later down the line. Unfortunately, the absence of periods means the health of the endometrium is impacted, but again this is not without hope. Introducing hormonal contraceptives to induce a regular monthly cycle can offset this risk by increasing the number of monthly periods, albeit in a contraceptive method.

There is an underlying genetic link suggesting that family history is a factor. This disease is also known to be associated with insulin resistance (insulin is used for the body to break down glucose to allow the body to use it for energy). Impairment to use or inability to produce insulin is what we know as diabetes type 1 or 2. The link is not fully understood scientifically speaking, but what is recognized is that women with PCOS have a higher risk of developing type 2 diabetes later in life, cardiovascular disease and gestational diabetes (temporary diabetes during pregnancy).

This insulin impairment contributes to weight gain, which further increases the risk of cardiovascular disease. However, understanding these associated risks and the fact PCOS has these links allows for women to make lifestyle changes that can certainly mitigate these risks.

PCOS being *associated* with these things does not mean the future of your health is written in stone. This is really important to realize because while there are associated risks, many of these are linked to multiple other factors including weight, cholesterol, genetics and lifestyle. Recognizing that your body has a link to insulin resistance and a predisposition to these things allows you to make informed choices about diet, lifestyle and exercise to regain some influence over them.

MANAGEMENT OPTIONS

PCOS behaves differently from many other period-related disorders, and so the approach for treatment is very different. As PCOS is often identified when fertility is in question, the treatment is usually directly targeted at achieving a successful pregnancy.

If we look at the shorter-term and longer-term problems women can experience with PCOS, this helps guide how treatments are considered:

Short-term problems

- Hirsutism causing personal distress – the high androgens affect the skin and hair, disrupting a person's quality of life, self-esteem and confidence.
- Weight gain and insulin resistance
- Fertility

Longer-term health issues

- Endometrial cancer risk
- Cardiovascular disease risk
- Type 2 diabetes risk

Your priority and stage in life at the point of diagnosis determines what treatments and interventions you may decide to take. It is common for someone diagnosed with PCOS at a time of facing fertility concerns to immediately launch into the fertility pathway of treatment. However, I would recommend also being mindful of the longer-term health risks beyond the fertility journey. I have seen women become diagnosed with PCOS who are then supported to have a pregnancy and then 'move on' without being aware of the need to be more health conscious due to the risks of their PCOS.

FERTILITY

Around 70–80 per cent of women with PCOS will have difficulty conceiving, but this is different from infertility and the majority of women will conceive naturally with the right support.

The main reason for infertility in PCOS is due to the lack of ovulation; the follicles are underdeveloped sacs and don't release an egg. Women have fewer periods and when they do menstruate these are often without an egg being released (due to the imbalance of hormones stopping the normal cycle from occurring). However, most women can become pregnant with the right treatment supporting them.

Many women can have their fertility supported without the need for assisted reproduction techniques (ART). There are medications available to help adjust the hormones and improve the ovulatory challenges. Losing weight can lower insulin levels and help adjust the hormones enough to restart a healthier ovulatory cycle – and even weight loss of 5 per cent can significantly improve the chances of success.

Clomifene

This is often the first treatment offered as it helps to stimulate ovulation. This works by targeting that brain-to-ovary circuit of the other ovary-stimulating hormones (FSH, GnRH and LH – see page 24). This circuit of hormones between the brain and ovaries is a complicated one: imagine the circuit of hormone messages going from the brain to the ovaries regulating the menstrual cycle. Ultimately, we want the ovaries to release an egg each month. In PCOS this circuit is blocked because too many messengers have disrupted the circuit and 'shut it down'. Clomifene comes in and redirects the circuit to allow the ovaries to be stimulated again and release eggs.

Clomifene is taken as a tablet once a day for five days early in the cycle to help encourage ovulation. Within three cycles, ovulation should have been re-stablished. Clomifene is often only given for six months; it can't be used for too long because it can overstimulate the ovaries, making it possible that the ovaries will produce multiple eggs each month and so there is a slightly higher chance (10 per cent) of twins.

Anything that interferes with the hormone balance will have side effects and clomifene is no exception: these are headaches, hot flushes, stomach pains and bloating and mood disturbances. There is a very rare side effect to which women being started on clomifene need to be alerted, which is called ovarian hyperstimulation syndrome (OHSS). This is a rare event that is also a risk within ART (IVF particularly) whereby the ovaries become overstimulated to a more severe degree. The stomach becomes incredibly swollen as the ovaries absorb too much fluid through swelling. Sudden weight gain, swelling, and shortness of breath are signs that urgent medical attention is needed.

Clomifene for many women, despite the side effects and rarer risks, can be all that is needed to help them become pregnant. The GP will also often advise losing weight: the weight loss causes insulin levels to drop and adding in clomifene can be a real success for achieving a pregnancy.

Letrozole

Often used to treat breast cancer, letrozole (also known as Femara) isn't licensed for PCOS but can be used with caution to stimulate ovulation. In cases where a drug was designed for one purpose but is also noted to help achieve something else, much of the research around it went into its primary purpose (in this case treating breast cancer), and so the risks and benefits aren't guaranteed for the secondary uses. In medicine we call this using the drug 'off licence'.

Letrozole is an aromatase inhibitor used to target the hormones in the wider tissues being converted by blocking certain enzymes. It works by stopping androgens being converted to oestrogen and this process tricks the brain into detecting a drop in oestrogen, thus producing more FSH (follicle-stimulating hormone), which is what is needed to stimulate the ovaries to release an egg.

Letrozole has less risks of multiple pregnancies compared to clomifene but because it is prescribed off licence, some GPs are less comfortable in using it.

Metformin

Used for the management of type 2 diabetes, its primary purpose is to lower insulin and sugar levels. While it is not licensed for PCOS, it is used more and more because of the wider benefits of managing the other PCOS symptoms of weight gain and disrupted insulin levels (thus reducing cardiovascular disease risks). The improvement in insulin levels can, in turn, help improve fertility. Metformin is also used for women struggling with PCOS who aren't concerned about fertility because of its benefit for the wider-spread symptoms. These women need to use extra contraception and be counselled for such because they don't immediately realize that while it is helping their other PCOS symptoms, it is also improving their fertility.

> ### Hirsutism
>
> Many women may feel uncomfortable going to their GP for help with male-pattern hair growth (on the chest, buttocks or face).
>
> This very sensitive symptom can lead to very real emotional distress. However, there are ways to treat hirsutism which can not only improve the physical symptoms but dramatically improve mental wellbeing:
>
> **Combined oral contraceptive pill** can not only help restore the menstrual cycle (albeit without ovulation) but the rise in oestrogen can help offset hair growth and loss, as well is mitigating endometrial cancer risks.
>
> **Anti-androgens** can lower testosterone levels to help with the hair growth (not suitable for use in pregnancy).
>
> **Spironolactone** is used for cardiac problems and is a mild diuretic which can have brilliant results for acne-prone skin, reducing hirsutism while overcoming hair loss and fluid retention. It cannot be used if trying to conceive or during pregnancy and can affect the salts in the blood (particularly potassium) so blood tests are needed to monitor.

PCOS and menopause

PCOS has an important pathway with menopause. When menopause rolls in, it doesn't erase PCOS entirely – but it does shift the landscape. The headline change is that the ovaries stop their chaos and the androgen levels (those nuisance male-based hormones) drop. For many people with PCOS this seems like wonderful news; symptoms like acne, oily skin and excessive hair growth subside because the hormones driving them fall. Cycles also stop becoming irregular because the whole system is winding down. It's the one time PCOS can't be blamed for unpredictable periods.

But menopause isn't necessarily a blissful reprieve from PCOS. While the ovaries go into retirement, there are still the other aspects of PCOS that continue – because PCOS is more than just a period disorder. The combination of natural ageing, reduced oestrogen levels and continued insulin resistance potential can escalate those other health risks such as weight gain, cholesterol and cardiovascular health. The high levels of androgens can remain elevated for some time and so there isn't an immediate relief from the hirsutism.

There are, of course, health risks associated with long-term exposure to hormone imbalances. The body is designed to have a status quo and too much or too little of anything can have a knock-on effect later down the line. Long-term exposure to low progesterone levels due to chronic anovulation in PCOS carries a risk of endometrial cancer. While menopause stabilizes things, being vigilant post menopause is still important. Any unusual bleeding or concerns must be investigated promptly by your doctor.

Hormone replacement therapy (HRT) is an option for people with PCOS and has a very valuable role in supporting the symptoms and changes that come with menopause. However, women with PCOS carry greater metabolic risks (such as cardiovascular disease and type 2 diabetes), which means their HRT options need adjusting in recognition of this. These health risks can also be mitigated with lifestyle changes such as improved diet and exercise.

So as women enter menopause and feel relief that the period-related chaos may seem to be over, the health risks associated with PCOS continue to be prevalent, if not even increased. If arriving in menopause at the natural age, this is also when those health risks for the general population begin to present themselves, but women with PCOS are already at a higher-than-average risk. Therefore, being mindful that weight, diet and lifestyle choices need even closer attention is necessary during this next stage of life.

PRIMARY OVARIAN INSUFFICIENCY (POI)

Primary ovarian insufficiency may sound daunting. A diagnosis of POI means that the ovaries are failing to produce eggs and thus deliver a regular and healthy menstrual cycle, therefore affecting fertility, at a young age.

POI can be a situation in and of itself – it happens spontaneously for an unknown reason or due to a genetic component and can be linked to early menarche, meaning our ovaries reach the point of retirement early because our periods started early. POI can also be the result of another disease or what we call *iatrogenic*, meaning caused by treatment for something else (such as chemotherapy or the early removal of ovaries).

Getting diagnosed

Exploring the *why* is the first part of the medical process. When women first notice periods becoming less frequent and dropping to below three to four times a year under the age of 40 then investigations are needed.

The diagnostic criteria for POI require that a woman is below the age of 40 and has reduced or absent periods for more than four months, along with an elevated FSH level in the blood. The high levels of FSH show that the body is trying to stimulate the ovaries, signalling that the dysfunction and core of the problem is the ovaries themselves. Checking levels over time shows the problem is not a temporary blip but the criteria for a diagnosis only requires a single blood test showing elevated FSH.

Causes of POI

POI can be a diagnosis of its own (primary) or as a result of other processes happening within the body (secondary). Understanding the cause dictates the response needed. However, ultimately there is no cure for POI, meaning treatments are often tailored to the body and consequences for the implicated health risks rather than addressing the underlying problem (depending on what this is).

Spontaneous

For some women, POI happens for an unknown reason and this can be difficult news to hear, which can inevitably lead to self-blame. Family history and genetics can play a part, so if the maternal bloodline has a history of POI or early menopause then this can be a factor.

Our ovaries have a finite number of follicles with eggs-in-waiting. Once these eggs are all used, the ovaries go into retirement. If we start our periods at an earlier age then we will deplete that reserve at an earlier age. Sometimes repeated cycles of IVF and assisted reproductive techniques that require ovary stimulation to quickly produce many eggs for harvesting can over time deplete our egg reserves faster than would have happened naturally.

Autoimmune

A big cause of POI is an underlying autoimmune disease process. Autoimmune premature menopause can happen on its own – the body's dysfunctional immune system has depleted the ovaries and induced POI. Or other autoimmune diseases can trigger POI as a secondary additional problem. Addison's disease is a classic example of an autoimmune disease whereby the main problem is a failure of the body to produce cortisol, but it also causes POI. Type 1 diabetes and thyroid disorders are other autoimmune conditions which can in turn lead to POI.

Iatrogenic

This term means 'as a result of medical intervention'. Sometimes medication or surgical treatments for one problem can lead to POI as an unintended consequence. If you are undergoing treatments such as chemotherapy, radiotherapy or the removal of your ovaries, it can lead to POI. It's important to weigh up benefits over risks in all treatments.

Other causes

Smoking, never having been pregnant and infections such as tuberculosis (TB) or mumps can also cause POI.

Management options

There is no cure for POI and so one of the first things to consider after diagnosis is processing the news emotionally. Beyond emotional support, management is aimed at the depletion of oestrogen and subsequent risks of early menopause, along with support for menopause symptoms.

Many doctors immediately discuss the medical support options available, but my experience as a patient (having faced POI through surgical menopause) is that I recognize this territory is a particularly emotive one.

Grief can arise with POI for all women, whether they have children already or not, and even if they had not planned to have children. Losing control of our fertility and hearing the words 'ovarian failure' can be very triggering. It is very important to recognize that disenfranchised grief is real and something to consider seeking emotional support for. Women can become angry, irritable and go through the motions of a grief response without necessarily recognizing that they are grieving. It is entirely normal and a valid response. Having an awareness of this and open communication with those around you is important to help with the healing process.

Hormone support

Early menopause is linked with so many period-related conditions, and POI is no different. The loss of oestrogen doesn't just cause menopause and the subsequent menopausal symptoms (which can be debilitating), it carries a risk of osteoporosis and increased cardiovascular disease.

Therefore, when POI is confirmed, women are encouraged to have hormone replacement therapy (HRT) to replace the oestrogen. There are different types, but if the uterus is still present then the combined contraceptive pill might be used to help reduce the risk of endometrial cancer. There is no 'first line' or preferred choice of HRT so this comes down to individual tolerance and needs (see Chapter 12 on pages 227–44).

Non-hormonal support

Bone protection is crucial with POI. Oestrogen is very much needed for our bone density and so it is recommended that women in premature menopause are screened using scans at timely intervals (influenced by individual risk) to assess bone density and monitor for signs of osteoporosis. Osteoporosis occurs when bones are weakened, which means easy fractures, shrinking height and a frailer body.

Bisphosphonates are a medication to help bone protection and can be discussed with an osteoporosis specialist.

Fertility

For young women for whom POI is spontaneous or the uterus is still present and healthy, there are still options for pregnancy. Sometimes if the onset of POI is detected early enough, ART to help harvest eggs may be explored, but it is not uncommon that fertility support is shifted towards utilizing egg donation. Some women donate eggs when they themselves are going through ART and have unused eggs following harvesting. These eggs are then fertilized with your partner's sperm or donor sperm and transferred to your own uterus. You can then become pregnant and carry a pregnancy and deliver a healthy baby yourself, but because the egg has been donated the baby will not be genetically linked to you.

Lifestyle and diet

To help protect from the longer-term health problems associated with POI, there are ways women can help themselves to reduce risks and feel better. Diet is very important and ensuring you are not depleted in vitamin D and calcium can help with bone health. Exercise, particularly weight bearing, also helps strengthen the bones, keeping osteoporosis at bay.

Smoking is bad full stop, but if ever there was a need for that final push to stop, this is it. Smoking already increases the risk of heart disease and osteoporosis and all those individual risk-increasing elements can compound, so anything you can do to reduce one risk can help.

CHAPTER SUMMARY

PCOS

To help with the wider body effects of PCOS there are other treatments to be aware of. There are multiple acne-targeting treatments, medications to help with weight loss and statins to help reduce cholesterol. It's also important to be aware of the overlap with insulin resistance; if this is the case it will become the main concern over issues with fertility, hair and weight.

When doctors tell women to adopt lifestyle changes, it can feel deflating or even condescending – but PCOS is one of those conditions where a small change can have impact (e.g. a weight loss of 5 per cent can significantly increase the chance of pregnancy and help mitigate other health risks).

POI

POI can have its impact on a woman's life overlooked. It is less prevalent than conditions like endometriosis or fibroids and depending on the cause there are no major symptoms of pain and heavy bleeding. But herein lies the problem: the resounding silence of no periods is a reminder of lost fertility and the onset of premature menopause. Sometimes the absence of symptoms is as profound as the presence.

Alternative ways of exploring having a family, although not the preferred option, do exist, as does support in managing the underlying cause and menopause. This is a condition where finding a community of understanding can truly help restore control, return confidence and reduce a sense of isolation.

Key takeaways

- Women can have polycystic ovaries *without having polycystic ovary syndrome*. The syndrome is diagnosed when there are polycystic ovaries with the presence of high androgens (male sex hormones) that can cause weight gain, hirsutism and other health problems including irregular periods.
- PCOS is a multi-system disease linked with insulin resistance and longer-term health risks, as well as fertility challenges. However, with the right treatments the prognosis for achieving a pregnancy is very hopeful.
- POI is rarer and has multiple underlying causes; but the implications for longer-term health risks needs to be recognized to make informed choices about HRT and lifestyle changes.

CHAPTER 12:
MENOPAUSE: MORE THAN JUST THE RETIREMENT OF OUR OVARIES

THE TRUTH ABOUT MENOPAUSE

Menopause deserves a chapter all of its own as it's such an important part of our journey with our periods. Menopause is the buzzword of the moment, and I have a personal love–hate relationship with this. On the one hand, we're finally acknowledging that this transition can bring major health challenges for *some* women. My concern is that the current online push, however well-intentioned, has led to exploitation by people without training offering courses or charging for unreliable, and in parts unsafe, information or supplements. My other concern is the portrayal that menopause is a catastrophic event that inevitably flattens every woman with its arrival. It isn't.

Here's the truth:

1. We absolutely need better education. Menopause was historically sidelined for all the usual patriarchal reasons, but education should not scaremonger.
2. The online space of health needs regulation and so my advice is to tread carefully. Much of what you need to support you during perimenopause and menopause is available for free from the right places.
3. Menopause does not have to be catastrophic or horrific – it can be a time of empowerment and even relief, especially if you have the right support.

I've been in menopause for about seven years now. It's been life-changing, yes, but I'm physically and mentally happier in a menopausal state than I ever was before.

Whether arriving at menopause surgically, chemically, prematurely or naturally, the impact is overarchingly the same. This means the support and options available are ultimately the same – entering menopause, like every aspect of period health, does not necessarily need to dominate your life.

Menopause doesn't need to be feared or confusing. Not everyone will struggle. If we strip away the noise and stick to the basics, women can be empowered and their confidence restored. The truth is there are many women, like me, not thriving *in spite* of the menopause, but thriving *because* of the menopause.

MENOPAUSE BASICS

Girls move from childhood into puberty. When a parent says their daughter is entering the teenage years, there's often an empathetic wince. That shift from hormone quiet childhood to hormonally active adolescence can be turbulent: acne, body changes, mood swings. Those years can be challenging for some, as teenagers must discover life with oestrogen, progesterone and the other fertility-orchestrating hormones taking over their bodies.

As parents we try to educate without catastrophizing, and we accept it as a transitional phase. We know, from experience, that some teenagers sail through these years while others wobble, but we rest easy in the knowledge that things will settle within a few years and that it is a transitional phase of life. We do not, as a society, overly medicalize this transition from one phase of life to another.

If puberty is the transition into our fertile years, menopause is the transition into fertility retirement. Whether we should medicalize this sparks debate. For many, it's a natural phase – like puberty in reverse. But increasing numbers of women enter menopause prematurely, often therapeutically for gynaecological disorders or due to treatment for cancer. For them, medicalization isn't optional; it's protective.

Part of the current advocacy surge exists because menopause used to be taboo. We prepared teenagers for puberty, but no one held a 'wellbeing session' for adults to say, 'Remember that rocky hormonal ride? You'll do it again, only in reverse.'

That's essentially menopause. As hormones shift, not always in a tidy straight line downward, their effects ripple through every system of the body.

Whether menopause arrives early or at the expected time, experiences vary. Some women glide through. Some feel overwhelmed by the magnitude of change. Most land somewhere in the middle: some turbulence, then adaptation. Whether you lean into herbal supports, meditation and embracing your silver streaks, or you use medical hormone therapy to smooth the edges, there is no single 'right' way.

What matters is understanding that these changes are hormonally driven; that support exists when it's too much; and that 'different' does not have to mean 'dreadful'.

TYPES OF MENOPAUSE

Many women don't realize that menopause itself is technically just one year: the 12 months after your final period. After that, you're post-menopausal. For simplicity I'll continue to refer to any time after the last period as menopause.

Perimenopause is the term used to describe the physical changes and transition into menopause – the hormonal autumn. Subtle shifts begin; cycles may change character, become lighter or more erratic; symptoms ebb and flow as the ovary-brain axis starts to wind down. Think of an engine low on oil: sometimes smooth, sometimes spluttery. This is like our bodies noticing the changing, declining hormones, the lack of egg follicles being stimulated and the body responding to this and changing accordingly.

- Perimenopause typically spans the late forties to early fifties (around ages 47 to 53), but many women notice symptoms in their early forties.
- Long-term contraception (e.g. the Mirena coil, other coils or the contraceptive pill) can mask perimenopause, so some women glide through largely unaware because exogenous hormones flatten the noise.

Menopause is marked by your last period, and the 12 months that follow. About 80 per cent of women reach menopause by age 54 (family patterns often run true, with a common range of 47–53). Post-menopause begins after that 12-month mark. Culturally, we tend to lump all of this under 'menopause', and for this chapter I'll stick with that for clarity.

> ### Red flag
>
> Once you've had 12 months without a period, any vaginal bleeding afterwards is not your period returning and must be checked. Benign causes like polyps are common, but post-menopausal bleeding can also signal endometrial cancer and should always be assessed by a doctor.

Early menopause (age 40–45)

'Early' simply means the transition happening between the ages of 40 and 45. It's a recognized variation and often tracks with family history or known health factors. It is not inherently alarming but worth noting so you can plan proactively.

Premature menopause and POI (under 40)

Below 40, menopause is considered premature – too early. Our bodies rely on hormones, particularly oestrogen, for our general health, strength and protection from diseases such as osteoporosis and cardiovascular disease (heart attacks and strokes). There are multiple reasons for a premature menopause, and an increasing number of women are falling into this category, which is why it is becoming more medicalized rather than being seen as a natural phase of life.

Returning to the changing seasons analogy, our bodies expect to transition gradually through the seasons and we might think of perimenopause as being a little like autumn, a welcome slowing from the intense heat of summer, before a smooth landing into winter (menopause). But if a blizzard suddenly arrives in spring this is too stark a change; our cells are not ready, leaving our bodies sensing that something is wrong.

Primary ovarian insufficiency (POI) has multiple underlying causes (see page 220) and should be investigated medically.

Surgical menopause

The removal of our ovaries is a sure-fire way of switching off fertility and putting the body from spring/summer into winter without the transition of autumn to ease the shift. There are different types of hysterectomy or oophorectomy, which are surgical procedures to remove different parts of our gynaecological organs:

- **Subtotal hysterectomy**: removal of the uterus, leaving ovaries and/or cervix intact. Does not induce surgical menopause if ovaries remain.

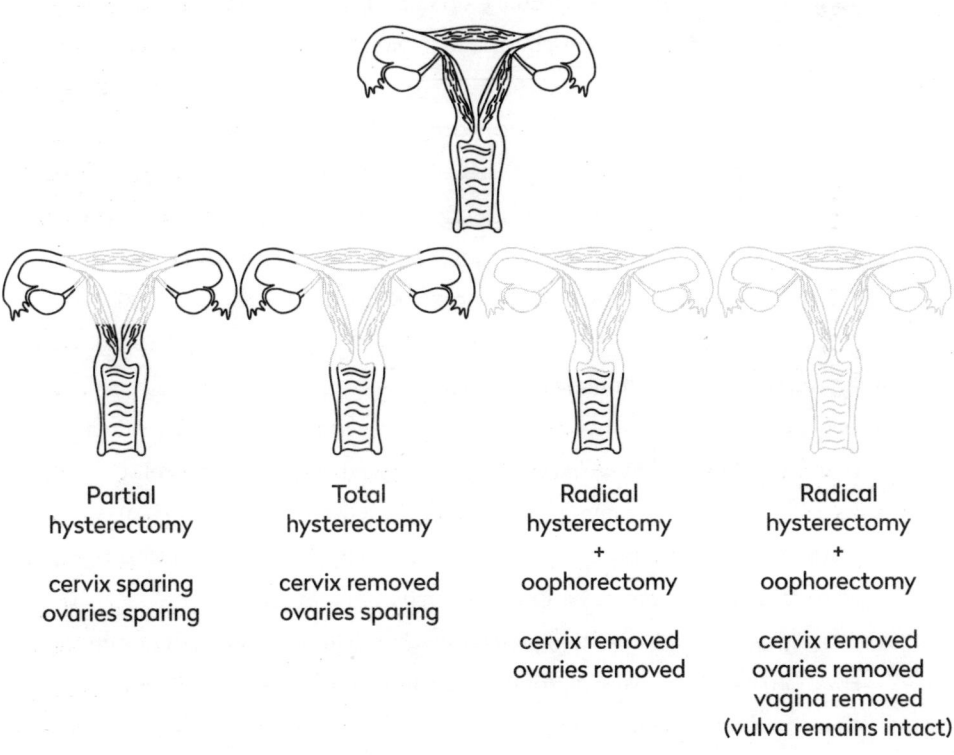

Partial hysterectomy

cervix sparing
ovaries sparing

Total hysterectomy

cervix removed
ovaries sparing

Radical hysterectomy
+
oophorectomy

cervix removed
ovaries removed

Radical hysterectomy
+
oophorectomy

cervix removed
ovaries removed
vagina removed
(vulva remains intact)

- **Total hysterectomy**: bilateral salpingo-oophorectomy – removal of uterus, ovaries, fallopian tubes and cervix. Does induce surgical menopause.
- **Oophorectomy**: removal of ovaries (often with fallopian tubes), uterus left in place. Does induce menopause.

These procedures may be carried out for cancer, risk-reduction in high-risk gene carriers, gynaecological disease such as endometriosis or adenomyosis or pregnancy-related complications.

Two crucial points:

1. If the uterus remains but ovaries are removed, you usually need progesterone alongside oestrogen when using HRT to protect the endometrium and reduce the risk of endometrial cancer.
2. Too many women are still not told clearly that removing ovaries leads to immediate menopause. This discussion should ideally happen prior to the surgery with adequate counselling and preparation for what to expect.

Chemical (medication-induced) menopause

Certain medications, most notably GnRH analogues/agonists (see page 159), temporarily switch off the brain-ovary signalling, inducing a *reversible* menopausal state. They're used in conditions like endometriosis and adenomyosis and in oestrogen-sensitive cancers to remove the hormonal 'fuel'.

- The onset is sudden: winter without autumn.
- In gynaecology, treatment courses are often time-limited (e.g. three to nine months) as a bridge before or after surgery or to gain symptom control.
- Experiences vary. For some (including me), the relief from endometriosis can feel like a heatwave replaced by cool snow. It is an immediate easing of pain that makes the vasomotor symptoms tolerable by comparison.
- For others, especially cancer patients who felt well pre-treatment, the abrupt addition of menopausal symptoms on top of chemotherapy side effects can be intensely challenging.

Whatever the method by which you have found yourself in menopause, the experience and symptoms of menopause are often the same. What becomes more pronounced is the absence of the perimenopause (a nice autumn preparing for winter), which can mean the stark contrast is a shock to the system.

IMPACT OF MENOPAUSE

During the perimenopause, symptoms tend to creep in gradually, like the slow turn of autumn leaves. But when menopause arrives abruptly, via chemical or surgical means, those same symptoms can hit within weeks, sometimes days.

We've all seen the cartoon version of menopause: a woman fanning herself at the window while everyone else sits freezing in jumpers. That caricature doesn't come close to representing the reality or distress these symptoms can bring.

Three things to keep in mind:

1. Symptom severity and duration vary wildly. Some women breeze through; others face years of chaos.
2. Symptoms can resolve naturally over time. Many symptoms fade after months or years without intervention.
3. For most symptoms, effective support exists, especially through HRT (hormone replacement therapy). Whether you choose to use it or not is entirely personal.

Someone once described menopause beautifully to me. She hadn't realized she was perimenopausal; her mood dipped, libido vanished, joints ached and fatigue took over. 'I thought I was losing my mind,' she said. And she isn't alone. I have even had many discussions over the years with women having profound life changes around the time of perimenopause, including an epiphany of sexual preferences. Women who previously identified as feminine suddenly felt more androgenous in their tastes and style. I even heard a remark that divorce rates peak around the menopausal age (although I'm not entirely sure how this could be objectively measured).

The takeaway? Hormones don't just regulate periods – they choreograph our entire being. Menopause, at its core, is not loss; it's transformation. How we respond and adapt remains in our control.

THE OBVIOUS SYMPTOMS

Hot flushes (hot flashes)

Some women call them flushes, others flashes – medically, they're vasomotor symptoms. A surge of blood flow causes sudden heat, sweating and sometimes palpitations or breathlessness. They can last seconds or minutes, often triggered by caffeine, alcohol or stress.

For some, it's a mild wave of warmth; for others, it's a full crimson tide creeping up the neck and face – often at the most inconvenient possible moment. I vividly remember sitting in a meeting, feeling that unmistakable flush climbing past my collar. Some episodes hide well under makeup; others might as well wave from across the table.

Night sweats

Same physiology, different timing. You wake drenched, hair plastered, sheets soaked, wondering if someone's spilt a jug of water in your bed (for those of us with small children, that's not always an irrational suspicion).

They're common in menopause but remember: new or worsening night sweats after years of stability warrant review. Persistent or late-onset sweating can signal other issues such as infection, thyroid change or even malignancy. Know your baseline and trust your instincts.

Libido and sex

It's easy to assume menopause means the end of sexual interest, and for some, libido does dip. But for others, it can genuinely improve.

There are multiple overlapping factors at play:

- **Hormonal shifts**: falling oestrogen affects vaginal tissue and lubrication, influencing comfort and desire.

- **Contextual shifts**: no pregnancy risk, greater self-knowledge and sometimes newfound freedom.
- **Physical shifts:** relief from previous diseases like endometriosis can eliminate pain and potentially make penetration or orgasm more enjoyable.

With the right support for vaginal health (see page 236), many women rediscover confidence and pleasure – even liberation. Menopause isn't the end of intimacy; it's simply a new chapter with a different manual.

LESSER-KNOWN SYMPTOMS

Skin, hair and joints

Oestrogen's reach extends to collagen, the protein scaffolding that keeps our skin supple, joints cushioned and hair strong. As levels decline, so does collagen. The result: thinner skin, fine wrinkles, easier bruising, hair thinning (especially around the temples) and those familiar morning creaks and joint aches.

Mood, memory and cognitive function

Our brains are studded with oestrogen receptors, especially in the regions controlling mood, focus and memory. When oestrogen dips, neurotransmitters like serotonin and cortisol wobble too. Cue irritability, anxiety, tearfulness, rage and the infamous brain fog.

It's not imagined, it's biochemical. For women juggling careers, households and hormonal chaos, this can feel like a betrayal of identity – especially when multitasking used to be your superpower. For those in premature menopause, it can be even harder: you're expected to be at your professional peak while your brain quietly rewires itself.

Energy, headaches and burning tongue

Energy dips, fatigue rises and headaches may increase – all common and manageable once recognized. Even the bizarre 'burning tongue' sensation, though rare, can be another side effect of hormonal fluctuation.

Insomnia

The body is exhausted but the brain wired, as if someone spiked your bloodstream with espresso. Up to 60 per cent of menopausal women experience insomnia.

Oestrogen plays a role in producing melatonin, the sleep hormone, so less oestrogen means less melatonin. The result is that cruel mismatch: daytime fatigue coupled with nighttime alertness. For many (me included), this can be more disruptive than the hot flushes.

The genitourinary syndrome (GSM)

With menopause comes a cluster of changes to the vulva, vagina and urinary tract, collectively called genitourinary syndrome of menopause (GSM) – though some clinicians still refer to this as GUS.

Because our urinary and reproductive structures sit so close together, hormonal changes in one affect them all. The classic symptoms include:

- Vaginal dryness and atrophy
- Vulval discomfort, itching or soreness
- Painful intercourse
- Urinary urgency or incontinence
- Increased urinary tract infections (UTIs)

As oestrogen and progesterone levels fall, glands produce less natural lubrication and the tissues become thinner, less elastic and more fragile. Pelvic floor muscles weaken, leading to leaks when sneezing or laughing. For women who've given birth or had gynaecological surgery, these changes can be more pronounced.

Reduced oestrogen also shortens and thins the urethra, increasing infection risk. Meanwhile, vaginal atrophy can make even gentle contact uncomfortable, sometimes leading to bleeding or recurrent infections such as thrush or bacterial vaginosis.

The good news? Local oestrogen therapy – in the form of creams, pessaries or rings – is extremely effective, safe and low-risk, even for many women who can't take systemic HRT.

Lichen sclerosis (LS)

The vulva goes through many changes during menopause, and knowing your vulva from your vagina is so vitally important at this time. The lack of collagen can make the skin become thin, fragile and prone to bleeding, and the autoimmune skin condition lichen sclerosis can become more apparent at this time.

Lichen sclerosis can masquerade as dryness or recurrent thrush. It's underdiagnosed, under-taught and potentially dangerous if missed. LS causes chronic inflammation of the vulval skin – thin, fragile, easily torn, often unbearably itchy. The condition tends to wax and wane, sometimes appearing in youth, quieting down, then re-emerging after menopause when oestrogen falls.

Lichen sclerosis is a pre-malignant condition which is far more common than people realize, and often missed because of:

- Cultural avoidance of using proper anatomical terms and women not knowing the difference between their vulva and vagina.
- Women being uncomfortable talking to the GP about these symptoms, let alone then letting the GP have a look 'down there'.

Chronic itching can often be mistaken for recurrent thrush or simply the vaginal atrophy changes. Women can have these symptoms for years and be totally unaware they have this condition. The problem is that if left untreated the skin undergoes changes of scarring and resorption of the inner and then outer labia, causing structural changes. Lichen sclerosis isn't just a fancy name for itchy skin; it is a premalignant condition with a risk of vulva cancer.

> **My story**
>
> While interviewing women for my charity podcast, *Mortal and Strong*, I spoke to a woman sharing her story of vulva cancer after years of being misdiagnosed with chronic thrush. Listening to her, I realized her story mirrored my own symptoms.
>
> Despite being a doctor, I'd never been taught about lichen sclerosis at medical school. I'd raised concerns with multiple clinicians about my own vulva soreness and had been told it was just menopause and sent away with lubricants. Years later, it took a gynaecologist to finally confirm what I already suspected, by which point scarring had begun and the changes were irreversible. That's why I speak about it now. Awareness saves vulvas and sometimes lives. Lichen sclerosis is something that commonly becomes more noticeable during menopause and because of its synergies with vaginal atrophy, is easily overlooked.
>
> If you have persistent itching, soreness or visible skin changes that don't improve with typical menopause treatments, ask your GP if it could be lichen sclerosis. Request a visual examination. LS can be managed with topical steroids, hormone creams and the right adjustments to hygiene routines, but without the correct management the potential for structural changes to the vulva tissue and malignancy are real, which is why it is important to not overlook something as seemingly minor as itching.

LONG-TERM HEALTH RISKS OF PREMATURE MENOPAUSE

There are two broad areas of the future that are impacted by premature menopause – our bone health and our heart/vascular health.

Bone health

Oestrogen is essential for bone turnover and keeping our bones strong and healthy. Women require this and are at much higher risk of osteoporosis than men because of the shift in hormones when entering the menopause. Osteoporosis is more than the visual of a lady with a hunched back leaning on a stick. Even with HRT, women can notice the shift in our joints and aches without our natural oestrogen. Our bone health is not just vital for our posture, but our health as a whole.

While osteoporosis isn't a threat to life, it impacts quality of life and can cause problems which can in turn pose a risk to life. Osteoporosis is a disease state where the bones have become weaker and more fragile. Aside from the shrinking height and posture changes, these brittle bones make a fracture far more likely. A trip or fall that once wouldn't have caused any problems can lead to a fracture, maybe one that requires surgery. Women with osteoporosis are at particular risk of fracturing their hips and needing a hip replacement. In the elderly population this in turn carries a high risk of secondary infections like pneumonia and can significantly cause a cascade of other medical problems.

Cardiovascular health

Oestrogen also helps manage cholesterol and blood-vessel elasticity. When it drops, the protective balance shifts. Women become more vulnerable to:

- High blood pressure
- Elevated cholesterol
- Atherosclerosis (narrowing of arteries)
- Heart attacks and strokes
- Type 2 diabetes

Lifestyle choices such as diet, exercise and stress management still play a major role, but without oestrogen's baseline protection, the margin for error tightens. This is where premature menopause does shift into needing a medicalized approach. While HRT is not the only solution for reducing risk, all available options (medications, lifestyle changes) need to be considered to invest in the longer-term outlook for menopause, not just the immediate hot flushes.

MANAGEMENT

I know that after reading through the symptom list, the idea of menopause can sound like a slow-motion car crash – flushed, sleepless, emotional, aching, forgetful and dripping in sweat. And yet I stand by what I said at the start: I actually do enjoy menopause.

Many of these symptoms may appear intense or arrive quite abruptly into your life but will settle down naturally on their own after a few months or years. They are not all there to stay. The mood fluctuations, hot flushes and some of the problems do settle down in time on their own. However, if the symptoms are too much or as a way of investing in your future bone and cardiovascular healthy, there is the very available and useful tool of HRT.

Hormone replacement therapy (HRT)

HRT is loved by some, feared by others and unfairly misunderstood by most.

Hormone replacement therapy has gone through different phases of adoration or deterrence over the past ten years. What HRT is, where it has a place and whether a woman needs or uses it requires a reflection on the benefits for not just symptoms, but the health benefits in terms of reducing the risk of those longer-term health implications of early menopause. A woman's right to use HRT remains just that – a woman's right.

HRT is the collective name for a group of medications used to replace the hormones no longer naturally circulating. Whatever the underlying cause of menopause, the loss of oestrogen and progesterone can cause unwanted symptoms, body or mood changes as well as health risks. The last of these is something often left out of discussion and we are not always good at doing what's right for the future in place of what we feel is right in the here and now.

Oestrogen is the central player within HRT as this is the hormone causing most of the problems. When the uterus is still present, progesterone must accompany the oestrogen to protect the endometrial lining and reduce the risk of endometrial cancer. For women who've had a hysterectomy, oestrogen alone may suffice.

- Removal of ovaries and uterus: oestrogen only required. *In endometriosis, progesterone is added to offset the oestrogen's influence on any residual endometriotic lesions.*
- Removal of ovaries but uterus remains: oestrogen and progesterone required

Delivery methods

How we replace the oestrogen is determined by what it is being used for. For overall ease of transition for women who are in surgical menopause prematurely, a systemic replacement is required – through oral tablets. For women entering menopause closer to the expected age, and for whom the need for oestrogen is to target specific symptoms like vaginal dryness, then vaginal creams or gels with oestrogen may be a preferred option.

How you take HRT depends on your needs:

- **Systemic HRT** (tablets, patches, gels): for general symptom control or premature/surgical menopause where body-wide replacement is needed.
- **Local HRT** (vaginal creams, pessaries, rings): for targeted relief from dryness or discomfort without systemic absorption.

Risks

HRT has spent decades under the microscope. Past studies created widespread fear after linking combined HRT to increased breast-cancer risk. Later reviews clarified the nuance:

- Yes, there can be a slight increase in lifetime risk with prolonged combined HRT (oestrogen + progesterone).
- Oestrogen-only HRT carries a smaller risk, sometimes neutral or even protective for certain conditions.

- The absolute numbers remain low and must be weighed against the much larger risks of doing nothing – particularly for women in premature menopause, where untreated oestrogen loss significantly raises the likelihood of osteoporosis and heart disease.

The reality: there is no universal rule. The right HRT is the one that aligns with your body, history and comfort level after informed discussion.

When HRT isn't an option

Not every woman wants to or can take HRT. Some women don't tolerate synthetic hormones, others simply prefer a non-medical route and a smaller number can't because of a medical reason to remove oestrogen. The key is understanding the trade-offs and focusing on quality of life.

So long as this decision is made with a full understanding of the longer-term implications (particularly on bone health and cardiovascular risk) what remains the focus of any management is restoring quality of life.

Alternative and complementary options

Diet and exercise

Early menopause means early risk for osteoporosis and cardiovascular disease, making this the best time to double down on physical health.

- Weight-bearing and resistance training strengthen bones and muscles.
- Cardio and flexibility improve heart health and mood.
- Prioritize calcium, vitamin D and omega-3s.

Supplements and herbal support

Calcium, vitamin D, magnesium and vitamin K2 all support bone health.

Herbal and 'natural' remedies – from soy isoflavones to black cohosh – have mixed scientific backing but can help some women. If they're safe and legal, and don't interfere with medication, they're worth exploring.

Vaginal health support

Even without HRT, you can improve vulval and vaginal comfort:

- Non-hormonal lubricants and moisturisers (many now formulated specifically for menopause).
- Condoms + quality lubricant can reduce friction and revive pleasure.
- Pelvic-floor exercises or physiotherapy to support urinary control and sexual function.

CHAPTER SUMMARY

I have demonstrated the full power and importance of oestrogen. That dominating influencer hormone dictating our periods and any consequent havoc, is certainly noticed when it is gone. The hormone some of us had a loathing for when it was fuelling the endometriosis or fibroid growth, now in its absence you can almost hear it smugly saying, 'Missing me now though, aren't you?'

Knowledge is so powerful in helping us to feel prepared for what to expect during all phases of menopause. The online space can be filled with alarmist stories of women's negative experience of menopause – my advice is to ignore the online noise and go to trusted sources of advice and listen to your own body and what works for you. While some of us may notice one or two changes, others experience the full spectrum and others still aren't really aware of what the menopause is or what to look out for. But the most important thing to know is that there is support available, including options such as HRT, and we shouldn't fear menopause.

Menopause can be a time of intense discovery and liberation and doesn't need to be met with apprehension and concern – because ultimately, we still have choices. It can be a poignant time for self-reflection and connecting with oneself again. Our life is, whether we realize it or not, in chapters – and while some elements are out of control it is us who writes the story ultimately.

I have met some women for whom the menopause has been the most liberating time of their life – the same goes for me. I know many women for whom the release from oestrogen allowed them to finally 'find themselves'. The influence of oestrogen on their mood, sexual preferences and monthly cycles had always felt almost unnatural or as if it was holding them back from something they couldn't quite explain. Without the influence of hormones shifting each month, they found mental clarity with stability, the confidence to recognize their true sexual preferences, or even sexuality. For many of us who have experienced painful or heavy periods for years, the chance to live without this monthly discomfort can also be liberating.

Key takeaways

- There are different paths for finding yourself in menopause:
    o Natural menopause
    o Chemically induced (through medications); often a short-term way of managing conditions like endometriosis and can be a welcome break from pain.
    o Surgically induced following a hysterectomy with the removal of ovaries.
    o Premature menopause through POI.

- Whatever the pathway for finding yourself in menopause, the effect on your health is not just the symptoms of hot flushes, insomnia and vagina dryness. There are many symptoms, but how these effect you compared to the next woman is variable and unpredictable. The important thing to know is that support *is available* whether in the form of HRT or other lifestyle changes.
- HRT is not just there for symptom relief; it can also help with bone protection (and staving off osteoporosis) and the risks of cardiovascular disease.
- There are multiple types of HRT and oestrogen replacement from tablets, creams and patches. There are many medically reliable places for support – navigate wisely but ultimately knowing there are options and this does not need to be a phase of life to be feared – for many it can come with freedom and empowerment.

CHAPTER 13:
THRIVING NOT SURVIVING

LIVING WITH A LIFE-CHANGING DISEASE

The body really is a remarkable, complex and often mystifying entity; as well as taking it for granted, at times we flit between having love, resentment or respect for all that it is and does. When things don't work the way we expect them to, it can be easy to feel that we've lost control of our identity or the ability to thrive. This absolutely does not need to the case with the right information, toolkits and support.

One of the biggest observations and revelations I have valued over my 20 years as both medical professional and patient is that there absolutely, always, without a doubt, needs to be a focus on thriving and not surviving. No diagnosis or life-changing health condition should be given the right to rob you of your identity or your right to *live*. Endometriosis took my uterus away from me, but it is not taking the essence of *who I am* or where I find joy in life. I know how, at times, this feels so beyond reach and almost an illusion for the lucky few. Don't get me wrong; there are days where I am far from thriving, but like a child learning to ride their bike, when we fall we pick ourselves up and start again.

To find a place of thriving over surviving requires the desire and the openness to receive the tools readily available to guide you. Living with a chronic illness is like living in a land prone to earthquakes or tornados; you can't escape the fact that another flare will occur at some point, but you have two options:

- Live among the wreckage, waiting for the next disaster; or
- Rebuild, savour the good days and keep your toolkit ready.

For each of the conditions outlined in this book we have discussed not only the symptoms but also the impact on fertility and our lives in general, and medical interceptions. Where medicine ends there can be an unspoken void of 'other' for most diagnoses. Recognizing this led me to found the charity Mortal and Strong (www.mortalandstrong.com) – because managing a major diagnosis is more than just medications or surgery, it requires a holistic approach to acknowledge and respond to every aspect of life that is impacted by a diagnosis.

It is one thing that our bodies have decided to rudely disrupt our plans for our life – but us women are strong and absolutely have the tools in our reach to dictate what our futures will look like. So here are those toolkits, the ones not written on a prescription by your GP. The toolkits can be described as social prescribing; recognizing the 'other' just as important aspects of a disease which – if responded to in the right way – help us to regain our womanly right to thrive not just survive.

> **To listen to your periods is to listen to your body communicating to you about your health.**

SPOON THEORY

If you have a chronic illness, you may have noticed how some days you have lots of energy but there is a limit on how much you can do before your body 'makes you pay for it'. Spending a full day out with the family seems to require more effort for you than it would for someone else, and you will probably return home needing a nap, or 'suffer' the next day or two as a result. Some days washing your hair seems like an insurmountable task because there's no fuel in the tank. *These are our spoons, influencing our energy reserve.*

When your body is in a state of inflammation, its reserve (physical, emotional, energy) is no longer what it was because it is trying to repair and deal with your underlying chronic health problem. In other words, you no longer have the fuel tank you once had. In the spoon theory your fuel tank is now replaced by spoons.

The theory goes that, for those of us living with chronic health problems, we have three spoons a day. On good days those spoons can stretch quite far and washing and drying your hair only uses one spoon, other days washing your hair can use up all your spoons and there is nothing left for anything else. If you use more than three spoons in one day, your body will need to replenish them, meaning you will likely need to nap, or the next day you start the day with only one or two spoons. You cannot use more spoons than you are given, or your body will make you wait until it restores that reserve.

This theory may come as a revelation, while for some it comes with a wry laugh or knowing smile. The spoon theory can not only help make sense of the fatigue and energy but also be a useful way of communicating to a partner, friends or family in a way they can understand. For me, some days the effort of doing the housework and having a shower will be the entirety of my three spoons. During summer holidays I must plan carefully; a day of busy activity with the children means the day after needs to be a home day to restore those spoons – because *for me* a day out all day uses more than three spoons so I am borrowing from the following day's spoon reserve.

Incorporating the spoon theory into your daily approach can be quite liberating. It is not a new restriction; it is something many women are already aware of and coping with. If this is you, you may even be struggling with a grief process and feeling frustrated about why your body can no longer 'keep up' with your previous busy lifestyle.

Your focus instead needs to shift from what you can no longer do to what you *can* do. It can be liberating to recognize that adjustments in planning your time, energy and reserve can let you do what you want to do – you just need to plan your spoons carefully. Earlier this year I took on the most physically demanding challenge I have experienced in many years. No, I didn't climb a mountain or run a marathon – I hosted an event for 10 days. I am 37 and for most people my age without health challenges their spoons would not have even been a factor or consideration as to how they could physically cope. I absolutely went into spoon debt by the end of the event, and it took me weeks, if not at least a month of rest, to replenish those spoons. But it was absolutely worth it.

The point with the spoon theory is that it gives you a way of communicating to those around you. It helps you check in with yourself each day to have an awareness of whether you are low on spoons or not. Listening to and consequently working with your body instead of forcing it to adapt to unrealistic expectations allows for more freedom. We can't change the underlying health challenges entirely, but we can change how we adapt and work with our body to regain our right to thrive.

THE GRIEF PROCESS

The spoon theory is a quirky way of acknowledging the new limitations imposed on us by our bodies. However, to live by it requires another process which can be harder: grief. The unspoken grief that comes with recognizing your body may have influenced your life in a way you weren't prepared for. Disenfranchised grief is a grief for which there is no card on a shelf to acknowledge, for which people don't send flowers and offer immediate empathy and support. The grief cycle of anger, bargaining, denial, sadness and finally acceptance is as real for someone processing a life-changing diagnosis as it can be for the loss of a loved one. It is entirely valid, and those emotions can come over days, weeks, months or even years.

Growing up, society and the media sold us a myth, a fairytale where we will find our happy ever after, with no preparation for the reality that our health may be interrupted at any age. There can be an illusion of fertility being a given as we make plans for our careers, our family desires and what we want for ourselves. When our body then presents chronic pain, inflammation, infertility and we face chronic fatigue, endless hospital appointments and days off work because of our symptoms, we begin to question those dreams we had made for ourselves. Suddenly the future we had planned seems an impossible fit for what our bodies are presenting. The natural emotional response is grief, and it isn't often talked about.

It is okay to have moments of anger at our bodies, others, the system. You may find yourself bargaining and trying 'just one more round of IVF' because the thought of resigning to the fact that you may not get that child you so desperately wanted feels too much. It can hurt, a very real visceral pain. This is grief, and although unpleasant, it is valid and it will pass.

Much like any other grief, the best way to process and heal to be released from its clutches is to talk, sit in it, explore those feelings. Communicating with those around you the reality of your grief and the *why*. Sometimes it can be a fear of a lost future – even if you are awaiting a prognosis the fear (for example of not being able to have children) can be there nonetheless; some days you unknowingly grieve for an outcome that hasn't even happened yet.

This is where having emotional support alongside some of these experiences is paramount in your healing.

MENTAL WELLBEING AND MICRO-TRAUMAS

When looking at challenges with our period health, we need to recognize the cumulative effect of the many ways it can impact our lives. Although some of these effects may be manageable on their own, when you add them all up, over time they can become overwhelming. You might have experienced the wild ride of hormone treatments, the fear and emotional response to your fertility being impacted, the mental toll of chronic pain and fatigue, the stress and worry of our work being impacted and the trauma of a loss of a pregnancy or surgery. One of those elements on their own would take its toll on your mental wellbeing, but everything together is like the Swiss cheese slices lining up and letting it all pass through.

Our bodies, mood and mental health do keep score. If you don't process something in a healthy way *in the moment* or very soon after, it resurfaces later on, seeking a resolution. If this happens repeatedly, these micro-traumas can cumulate, causing a bigger issue for your mental wellbeing. Intervening early can make all the difference. Sometimes simply explaining what you are going through (grief, micro-traumas, spoon theory) to those around you can profoundly change their support, patience and understanding. Masking through the journey, pretending that everything is fine, can be a slippery slope.

Sometimes the relief of taking the mask off – having a day to process, cry and feel the reality of what you are experiencing – is enough in itself to help heal those micro-bruises. And having the humility to seek support at the right times can be a major-investment in your future. If you and your healthcare team recognize the potential impact that your diagnosis and symptoms can have on your mental health and you get the right support, it will be much more bearable.

> **My story**
>
> One of the worst aspects of the years spent battling with infertility, diagnosis and treatment for endometriosis and the miscarriages – far worse than the pain – was the mental toll. The silent lurker that crept upon me gradually like a slow fog that I did not see coming. The unprocessed, unresolved emotional bruises of those micro-traumas that I felt I could handle and move on from (keeping focused on the end goal of being well, with a pregnancy and endometriosis managed) all returned at once and landed with PTSD (post-traumatic stress disorder) and severe PND (postnatal depression).
>
> Having never had a significant history of mental health issues, this came as a shock (I had been on a low dose of serotonin-based medication for many years but had not had what would be considered a major mental health episode or difficulties). Despite the repeated miscarriages and IVF attempts, as well as the toll of cycles of hormones and other treatments for my various health conditions, no medical professional ever offered emotional support. Not once. I cried in every single midwife appointment, but still no one said a word. (I have since been fortunate to address this issue systemically in working with new training programmes for regional midwifes, reiterating the importance of earlier intervention and recognizing the red flags for mental struggle.)
>
> The pregnancy was complicated by an undiagnosed fibroid, causing bleeding and an irritable uterus. After all the miscarriages, I was told to expect to lose the pregnancy. After I hit 24 weeks suddenly the shift was to push me as close to 34 weeks 'because it was safer for the baby'. By 30 weeks I was admitted on bed rest because of the bleeding and contractions. Then came a traumatic emergency caesarean section at 34 weeks; I nearly died and my son needed resuscitating twice.

All those unprocessed micro-traumas came together and this final one was the 'straw that broke the camel's back' and I mentally broke. I landed in the darkest place I didn't know could exist and it was beyond frightening. Worse still, it was all completely preventable.

Had someone said to me at any of those junctures to even *try* seeing a therapist, whether I needed it or not – had someone sat me down to say, 'take a pause – let's just process some of these things for a moment'. It would have forced me to withdraw from the closet of my brain those micro-traumas I thought I could brush aside and move on from. In my hyper-focus of getting 'well' and getting pregnant, I neglected my mental wellbeing.

I share this as a worst-case example. One of the most important things I'd like to iterate in this chapter is to encourage you to seek support for what you are going through emotionally as this must be considered alongside the management of what you are going through physically. The two are very much interlinked but prescriptive medicine will often focus on one and not the other. It is therefore upon *you* to have an awareness of this and approach these journeys with a consciousness of just how vital mental wellbeing is.

RELATIONSHIP IMPACT

Whether a spouse, a partner, a family member or friend – the impact on our relationships, particularly intimate ones, can all be affected.

Support is often delivered to you, the patient, and you are undoubtedly the one very much 'in the thick of it'. But as you process and react to these health challenges, a degree of burden also falls upon whoever it is standing behind you. Often these experiences have a way of strengthening our relationships and uniting a couple as they navigate the journey together. But in some cases, it can create rifts and tensions and expose subtle fractures in our relationships, and not everyone makes it.

From what I have seen both as a doctor and patient, there are multiple things that can influence how much your condition can take a toll on your relationship. If your own emotional wellbeing and support systems aren't in place, it can be tempting to purge those unresolved emotions and micro-traumas through outburst, hostility and emotional dumping onto a partner. The tension becomes palpable for both and suddenly your relationship can feel under threat. This is not to say this won't heal or restore in time — but allowing space and communication as a couple is crucial.

Many women will research and gather as much community support as possible and become immersed in this world of fertility, endometriosis or diagnosis. They find common ground and connection with people 'who get it'. It is important to relay these insights and information learned to your partner so that they don't feel left on the outside and are equipped with the tools to support you. In an ideal world your partner would do their own research to understand how to help you, too. However, remember that no one will dive deeper into the rabbit hole of understanding like the person experiencing the challenges first hand, and so patiently relaying what you discover and explaining what you need from them can be a relationship lifeline.

The best advice I ever heard from another GP during the thick of heightened stress within our own household was that it's okay to pretend that it's not happening from time to time. Life can become all-consuming with hospital appointments, fertility injections, venting about the pain and work stresses. Without realizing it, everyday dynamics begin to orbit around your diagnosis and health – this is neither sexy nor romantic and doesn't often allow for intimacy or even a much-needed hug. Taking time to pause and put a temporary embargo on any discussions of what is happening in life, to pretend for an hour, an evening or even day, can be another relationship lifeline. Have a code word to gently remind one of you that for one evening no one is to mention anything relating to the embargoed topic. Watch a film, have a meal. Remember what life was like without all these stresses and challenges. Force yourself back into a state of normalcy. It isn't masking so much as temporarily providing release from the cortisol-driven fight or flight state. It allows mental and physical breathing space from those micro-traumas. It invites in the opportunity and permission to laugh and forget. The benefit to the mind, body and relationship can be immensely powerful.

ADVOCATE USING ICE: IDEAS, CONCERNS AND EXPECTATIONS

The ICE method is taught to doctors in training to effectively derive information from patients:

- **Ideas**: what you think the underlying problem is. For example, you are reporting painful periods and you suspect you have endometriosis.
- **Concerns**: what you are worried about. For instance, you are worried that if you have endometriosis there will be an impact on your fertility and the pain is so extreme you are worried there may be a degree of organ damage.
- **Expectations**: what you are hoping will be agreed from today's appointment. You may simply want reassuring or you may be expecting a referral to a gynaecologist for investigation to check for endometriosis.

All UK-trained doctors are taught this communication tool during medical school. Unfortunately, with time pressures, etc. many forget its value once set loose on the wards as a licensed doctor, but they will recognize it once you start speaking in this way.

These three simple words help you to both speak the same language simply, effectively in a way both you and your doctor can understand. Sometimes even using the key phrases 'my ideas are' or 'my concerns are' can trigger the doctor to tune in and recognize what you are communicating. It allows for a non-confrontational two-way communication that provides autonomy and validation for the patient. The doctor may hear your expectations are for a referral, but this communication style can allow them to respond and explain why that referral may not be needed right now.

I used to struggle at times myself as a patient to feel heard and understood. Then one day I realized that I wasn't using this communication tool despite having been taught it as a doctor. The next time I was met with resistance by a doctor, I felt the frustration rise and thought – let's give this a go. I calmly asked:

'Please can you document in my notes what my ideas, concerns and expectations were today?' I swear that in that moment, the doctor's face changed and it was like she could suddenly understand me. The entire consultation shifted, there was no tension or conflict and she *heard me*. Instantly we found a mutual place of what my ICE was and what she wanted to do as the doctor – the outcome was the best clinical response to both.

SELF-HELP

Research

Health education equips patients with autonomy, control and empowerment. Doing your homework and gathering information is paramount to becoming empowered with the tools to navigate, manage and thrive beyond whatever havoc your periods may be trying to cause you.

My advice is to scroll safely. There is so much misinformation online, with facts being warped for clickbait; personal opinions and experiences being presented as warnings or guidance. I have even seen patient advocates producing 'patient information' booklets without any formal qualifications. A diagnosis does not a qualification make, and while patient advocates sharing their story can be wonderful for providing community support and shared experiences as insight, these are not the sources of reliable, medical information.

Look for the PIF Tick on online health information – the Patient Information Forum is the UK's only regulator of online health information to ensure the content has been produced by trained professionals to ensure reliability, authenticity and safety. It is not currently a legal requirement, but most responsible health educators and organizations have committed to the regulatory process, me included.

Diet

I get asked about this a lot and my personal answer is yes – diet does have a role in personal health and wellbeing. This comes back to the reality that we are primal beings and we have evolved so that our cells, proteins and enzymes rely on what we ingest to function properly. Too much of the wrong things, or not enough of the right things, absolutely upsets our systems.

There is much discussion of anti-inflammatory diets within the endometriosis community particularly. More and more light is being shed on to the link between certain food groups having an inflammatory trigger to them, i.e. that eating certain foods can raise our body's inflammatory state. With conditions like endometriosis and adenomyosis, we have too much inflammation happening in a dysfunctional way and we want to dampen that inflammatory state, not fuel it (this is a very simplistic explanation of how the anti-inflammatory protocols work). My caution and personal belief with this is that extreme diets of any kind can leave the potential to miss essential food groups that our bodies need. It is something I advise exploring, with caution. My personal approach is that I try to eat as simplistically and 'close to nature' as possible by ensuring the core food groups are consumed and avoiding processed foods, but having a balanced approach. I even explored Ayurvedic diets and saw a resonance for me personally. Through exploring these different valuable connections between diet and my own body's response, I did notice certain food groups that I personally need to avoid.

My advice would be that looking at your diet, for any health condition, is always a valuable starting point. Keeping a food diary with symptoms (there are some great apps to help with this) can help you spot potential triggers, potential imbalances of too much or too little of one food group. Explore the autoimmune diets (from reliable sources). I personally never go for an extremist protocol that eliminates essential nutrients, but there is a lot to be said for having an understanding of what foods can be pro-inflammatory, and thus useful to reduce or avoid when you are trying to reduce inflammation. In endometriosis, for instance, you have too much unhelpful inflammation happening. There are many foods that people don't even realize could encourage this unwanted inflammation, including particular vegetables or meats. Small changes here could massively improve symptoms and I know I have seen it in myself and other women. There are also brilliant nutritionists who can help – look for their qualifications, experience and regulatory processes to ensure you find someone you can trust with your health.

Emergency toolkit for flares

When a flare arises you can be overcome with pain, emotions or fatigue. In that moment trying to articulate to a partner what you need or even having it available for yourself isn't always feasible. When you are feeling *well*, prepare an emergency toolkit to have ready for the next flare and communicate it with someone close to you. This could be a box containing the right pain relief, a heat bag, a nice candle and book for comfort, your favourite jumper and some chocolate. This is a toolkit of practical and emotional necessities to help you that is there ready when you need it. As part of this preparation, explaining to your partner what you want from them when you are in a good place is far easier. During a flare you may want a cuddle, or to be left alone. This is not always easy to communicate when in the midst of pain at a score of ten, and what can sometimes happen is an attempt to communicate comes out as an emotional outburst, failing to achieve the desired effect. Communicating and preparing *when well* means the tools are there ready when you need them.

Community of support

Finding your tribe is so important to avoid the potential for isolation. There is nothing like being able to offload and share with people who can relate and understand. The online community space is incredible for this. The validation and recognition of knowing you are not alone can relieve so much burden and emotional stress. Rabbit holes of humour, supportive memes and relatable videos can help carry you through the journey without feeling alone and can have a significant beneficial influence on your journey. Being able to support others in turn can also build your confidence and sense of purpose.

> ## Neurodiversity
>
> Neurodiversity has a very important role within period health (see page 117). Anyone with confirmed or suspected neurodiversity – particularly attention deficit hyperactivity disorder (ADHD) and, to a lesser extent, autism spectrum

disorder (ASD) – will already realize that your experience of symptoms, treatments and anything that has an ability to influence mood has a more significant impact.

People who are neurodiverse, ADHD particularly, can often be more sensitive to mood changes – they can feel deeper, stronger and sometimes even be overwhelmed by the degree of these emotional changes. This is why people with ADHD are more susceptible to PMDD (see page 56) – that emotional dysregulation can be more marked. This means any period disorder that requires hormone treatments, which can upset the status quo of emotions, needs a greater degree of understanding. My advice for people querying or confirmed to have ADHD: it is even more important to recognize what hormones trigger what mood changes. High progesterone in ADHD has a stronger potential for inducing anxiety and dark, unpleasant thoughts. This may be helped by oestrogen-based hormone treatments, or even by GnRH analogues (see page 159). Conversely, progestogens may make these anxiety and low mood spells worse. Again, what works for one person won't be true for someone else. One person with ADHD might do really well on the combined oral contraceptive pill, whereas for someone else that might cause too many mood changes.

Tracking your cycle, your mood and noting what hormone treatments have worked (or not worked) is a really useful tool for someone with ADHD or neurodiverse tendencies. You are not 'going crazy' if you find these profound shifts in hormones harder to tolerate than someone neurotypical (and this might be the first time you are discovering that hormones have a stronger role for neurodiverse individuals). But there is hope. It is important to know that being neurodiverse has the potential to mean the shifts in hormones with pregnancy, postpartum (increased risk of postnatal depression), menopause and hormone treatments could be more profound and have a greater effect on mood. This knowledge allows for preparing, doing your research to avoid potential pitfalls and communicating to your friends and family.

More and more research is beginning to spot an overlap with neurodiversity, period disorders and connective tissue diseases (hypermobility) and even POTS (postural orthostatic tachycardia syndrome). This is leading to a potential genetic link and in time could lead to more directed treatments.

Retaining your identity before your diagnosis

The final item on this doctor's prescription list is to remember that beneath the heavy periods, painful periods, hospital appointments, community spaces, memes, booklets and injections, there is a woman who at one point had a life and a vision of herself. Who is she and where is she right now? That young girl you once were who felt like that first period was a life-changing event maybe didn't know what was coming for her. But what would you want her to know and how much of her life, your life and who you still desire to be is a priority? Because this is the point, isn't it? Right at the start of this book I wrote about how our periods are part of us as reproductive beings. The chapters in between – on the potential complications and the stages of your life with pregnancies or losses, tests and surgeries – these are just that: chapters. They do not define the whole book that is you. Remember that you are a woman with a desire to thrive, live and find joy in the world – this is still available to you and needs to remain the primary focus of any steps moving forwards. Your diagnosis does not define you. First and foremost, you are a woman whose identity and right to live do not need to be dictated by your periods.

CHAPTER 14:

ARE YOUR PERIODS HEALTHY AND HAPPY?

I began writing this book by establishing some grounding principles for what should constitute a healthy period. Within these foundations is my personal preference for avoiding use of the word 'normal' with reference to period health due to concerns over its historic use in describing painful and heavy periods. Because painful and heavy periods are far from normal. Period.

Through these pages you have humoured my analogies and metaphors, rogue as some may have been, as I have tried – in as much depth as your period health deserves – to equip you with the knowledge to reclaim ownership of your life. We have covered the fact your eggs were there in your mother's uterus, the obstacles that can stop them from finding their own potential sperm for conception, how the hormones oestrogen and progesterone not only conduct our menstrual cycle but also our behaviours and motivations.

So much of our physical and emotional experiences at every stage of life are influenced by our periods, those periods being a marker of our reproductive selves and the core of what we as primal mammals are designed to do (i.e. reproduce). And so much of what can go wrong within our gynaecological organs can be dictated by our genetics. Issues and disruption can be infuriatingly slow to present and complex to manage.

Much information is contained within these pages. I hope that I have debunked some myths and corrected a skewed landscape of period health to return control of your period health to you. As both doctor and patient I recognize that true autonomy in decisions about our health only comes through being equipped with all the information. I have learned the hard way that not all doctors are taught about how these diseases work to a specialist level; it is no wonder patients are feeling lost when in their short consultations they are inevitably not being presented with enough information to truly be autonomous and empowered.

To complete this book, I will finish with some of my own pitfalls, to reiterate the key aspects I believe commonly affect many women. I truly hope the following may serve as a final take-home pearl of wisdom.

WHAT DO I WISH I HAD KNOWN THEN THAT I KNOW NOW?

We understand pain as a warning signal that something is wrong, but in endometriosis these signals are misfiring

For so long I felt dismissed and ignored and became increasingly anxious because the pain I was in was so severe, yet the doctors were simply offering me more and more pain relief. Why didn't they want to explore what was happening or take another look?

No one properly explained to me that in endometriosis the pain felt is not proportionate to, or a marker of, the disease activity. The pain receptors become hypersensitive to oestrogen, meaning that in the absence of a cure it was more than appropriate to find other means of silencing those pain receptors. I really wish this had been drilled into me because I would have complied much more had I realized this. Instead, I felt I had to 'stay in tune' with the pain in my own misguided belief that in doing so I was monitoring the disease activity. I could have saved myself years of needlessly suffering.

There is no cure for endometriosis

I knew this, but I never fully grasped the concept of what this meant in terms of living with a lifelong incurable disease. For many incurable medical diagnoses, this news is delivered with adequate counselling and support to understand the implications moving forwards, but this is not the case with endometriosis. Had I grasped this fully I would have realized earlier that I should be prepared for the eventuality of a hysterectomy and I would have re-orientated my expectations that any treatments were likely not going to cure my pain. Had I had more realistic expectations this could have allowed me to explore wider means for support earlier on, sought counselling and communicated the impact of this life-changing diagnosis to those around me. Instead, I was on a turbulent spiral of hope and disappointment and had little autonomy in my own care.

Not all gynaecologists are endometriosis specialists and for advanced disease stages (stage three or four) your care should be managed by an endometriosis specialist centre

This was the kicker that took me down a path of being left without treatment for a year longer than I should have, causing organ damage, and saw me being advised to pay privately for IVF that was never going to work.

IVF (or any type of ART) has its place for many organic disease processes that affect infertility

But it should not be rushed into without the right support and guidance by your specialist gynaecologist where appropriate.

Hormones impact us as human beings far beyond the timing of our monthly periods

They dictate the essence of our desires, behaviours, energy, mood, ambitions. Understanding and recognizing this is important when introducing hormonal treatments, especially when transitioning into an induced menopausal state that will consequently impact more than just our gynae health. This truth is not shared to be alarmist, quite the opposite – knowledge allows for far better-informed choices in what hormone treatments are suitable for us. Had I recognized earlier that I was personally very emotionally sensitive to synthetic progesterone (progestins) it would have greatly changed how I approached the treatment options in my own journey.

Menopause introduces a whole new phase of life for a woman, physically and mentally

While this shift can be premature because of an underlying gynaecological disease, this doesn't need to be feared. When equipped with the right information and help, we have choices that allow us to regain control over our bodies and support us through the symptoms. I am loving being in menopause because I have found such comfort in its emotional stability and in being free of pain and aggressive disease.

WOULD I HAVE DONE ANYTHING DIFFERENTLY?

Hindsight brings both regrets and wisdom but changes nothing in the end. I cannot say where, if I knew then what I know now, anything would have changed for better or worse for me. What I do know is that information is not readily shared with women, meaning their ability to navigate these very prevalent period-related challenges is restricted. This is why I have written this book. Because while I realize looking back serves no helpful purpose for me, the reflections upon my journey as both doctor and patient have allowed me to identify some very real failings in the system, in communication and within our culture. Change is happening and discussions on period health are far beyond what they were 20 years ago.

I was always destined to have a rocky road with my endo. While the journey could have been vastly improved for me had I been counselled the way patients should be with such a diagnosis, I recognize that entering menopause was always going to be the step that provided me with the most relief.

I do feel that had I been equipped with even some of the knowledge within this book, I might have avoided a couple of miscarriages, avoided paying for IVF that was never going to work and been a better patient in taking any pain relief offered to me. My relationship may have been stronger with adequate emotional support and understanding as we experienced those micro-traumas without awareness and healing. Counselling for women given a major diagnosis like endometriosis, particularly in light of how complex a disease it is, is something which I feel should become part of the management pathway. In the absence of that, the best we can do is educate ourselves, our daughters and those around us.

The question should not, therefore, be around what I would have done differently; instead, it should focus on what I wish had happened earlier on. Many might expect me to say, 'Get diagnosed earlier', but no. A diagnosis without information and explanation is as pointless as a diagnosis without management. *Understanding* the disease – its implications, the management and support options – forms the basis of empowerment, improved quality of life, control, mental wellbeing and, ultimately, the ability to thrive despite the disease, not just survive with the disease.

WHAT DO I WANT MY DAUGHTER TO KNOW?

I sit with a very bizarre sense of reflection writing this book. As I settle into post-menopausal life, still with the lingering complications of endometriosis in my pelvic organs (what's left of them), my daughter is entering puberty herself. I can recognize cyclical cramps beginning and know that the arrival of menarche in our house is on the horizon. Last month she was doubled over with a hot water bottle, complaining to me how it is 'so unfair' that girls must go through this and not boys. I half laughed, half looked on with fear and apprehension. My first thought is to ensure that I, as her mother, can advocate on her behalf until she is an autonomous adult, as I have a duty to make sure I equip her with the knowledge and tools she needs.

There is a scene in the *Hunger Games: Catching Fire* film (spoiler alert) where the lead character is finally over the trauma of the first film, sinking into a naive sense of peace, thinking the challenges are 'all behind her'. Plot twist and she discovers she must re-enter the warzone and 'do it all over again'. Her face as she falls to the floor in disbelief captures how I, as a mother of a teenage daughter beginning to show signs of disproportionate period pain, feel. *Not again.* I, like anyone else, do not have a crystal ball. While genetics and family history are undoubtedly influential, all I can do is be mindful rather than hyper-vigilant or premature in taking her to the doctor demanding investigations.

Instead, my mission is to equip her with the knowledge and insight that I never had and support her on her journey.

By presenting this book, I am openly challenging our school education system to do better – for too long girls and women have not been educated adequately about period health and this is a huge injustice. There is so much knowledge and insight that still is not covered on the school curriculum. So, I am absolutely aware of my responsibility as her mother, a mother with experience, to find a balance of educating her as and when needed so that she is equipped and confident in managing her period health as she enters her own reproductive years.

THE FUTURE FOR PERIOD HEALTH

I realize that as I sit and write this book, scientists somewhere are diving deeper into the cellular core of what is happening with some of these diseases, endometriosis particularly. I sit with eager anticipation, watching the research field longingly. While this research will no longer help me, I know how much it will have an enormous impact on so many other women. The focus is finally shifting from looking at endometriosis as purely a hormone-driven disease to gaining better understanding of the inflammatory processes behind it. Trials into new treatments and management approaches have already begun and I have such hope and confidence for this direction. I look forward to the day when I write the updated version of this book which will provide even greater depth and hope for so many women.

THE IMPORTANCE OF HOPE, JOY AND THE PRIORITY TO THRIVE

The minute you start working with your body and listening to what it *can do*, everything changes. You regain control over your life and ability to thrive, not just survive. Our periods may dictate the essence of us as reproductive beings, but they do not have the power to dictate us as living beings – not when we are equipped with the right tools.

I have experienced first-hand how profoundly health issues can cause ripples that impact relationships, work and mental wellbeing. They doesn't need to, though.

But if they do or have, there remains hope. There is always hope. Wherever you find yourself currently, the ability to take a pause, take a breath and reflect is always there. One thing I have learned from another wise woman is that we as women are very good at *'shoulding'* all over ourselves. *'I should be able to still work full time,' 'I should be able to have children,' 'I should be able to maintain a tidy home, have a social life, have sex three times a week.'* These *'shoulds'* are the inner voices within our heads put there by society and cultural habits, mixed with our desires for a life we want for ourselves.

We absolutely have the right to desire and to dream, and aspirations are what carry us forwards. Where we unknowingly create more hurdles for ourselves is when we refuse to acknowledge the limitations beyond our control and continue, with increasing exhaustion, to hammer that square peg into a round hole. Sometimes to admit defeat and recognize some of those *'shoulds'* aren't feasible, is to regain control and be released from a futile expense of mental and physical energy.

I cannot physically climb a mountain with all the will in the world; my hips do not allow it. I could stay bitter, train and push my body to the extreme in a mental battle because of an inner sense of entitlement that at 37 I *should* be able to. I trained for five years and worked for ten as a doctor and was fiercely passionate and had so many career aspirations laid out for myself. *I should* have been able to continue to do the job I loved. But my body is not what I thought it would be. Fighting that and pushing it for too many years in a reluctance to accept these facts led to depression, anger and resentment at my body and situation. The moment I stopped *'shoulding'* on myself and shifted the *should* mindset to *can*, everything changed. Instead of hammering a square peg into a round hole, I changed the shape of the hole.

Recognizing what I can do opened up a new world and life for me. Finding hope by listening to those around me who were beacons of light navigated me through to a place of post-traumatic growth that was a genuine lifeline. Microtraumas, traumas and experiences don't need to keep hold of us in a dark place. The strength that we find by moving forwards beyond those experiences can be profound and powerful. Someone once said to me: 'You will find a strength you never knew existed.' I found it difficult to believe those words in that moment, but I dared to hope. I listened, I trusted and I let those words lead me forwards.

By accepting what I can control, what my body can do and stopping *shoulding* – I reclaimed control over my life and found new joys in ways I had never imagined before. The principles of this apply to any health challenges and became the basis for the charity I founded. Strength is not something we immediately have: it is proven in the transcendence from our hardest challenges. Using hope to guide us, focusing on the joy that makes life worth living, fuels strength and shifts us from survival mode to thriving.

GLOSSARY

ABLATION A procedure that destroys the uterine lining (endometrial lining) to reduce heavy bleeding. Can impact future fertility.

ADENOMYOSIS A condition where tissue similar to the endometrial lining grows inside the muscular wall of the uterus. Causing heavy, painful periods and a 'boggy' uterus.

ADHESIONS Bands of scar-like tissue that can form after inflammation, infection or surgery. Often seen in endometriosis.

AMENNORHOEA The absence of periods. Primary amenorrhoea is where a woman has never had periods; secondary amenorrhoea is when a woman who previously had periods experiences them stopping.

ANDROGENS Male hormones, such as testosterone.

ANOVULATION A menstrual cycle without the release of an egg. Common in PCOS, causes irregular cycles, fertility challenges and low progesterone levels.

ART (Assisted Reproductive Technology) The term used for fertility support using interventions such as IVF or IUI.

ATROPHY (vaginal) Thinning, drying and inflammation of the vaginal tissues due to low oestrogen, often experienced in menopause. Can cause pain, irritation and recurrent urinary tract infections (UTIs).

BREAKTHROUGH BLEEDING Unexpected bleeding (period) while on hormonal contraception.

CERVIX The neck of the uterus, the entrance, which opens slightly during ovulation and periods, and dilates for childbirth. Sits at the top of the vagina and allows sperm to enter the uterus for fertilization during intercourse.

COMBINED CONTRACEPTIVE PILL Oral tablets containing oestrogen and progestogen (synthetic progesterone). Regulates cycles, treatment used for period disorders and as a contraceptive.

DYSFUNCTIONAL UTERINE BLEEDING (DUB) A term used to describe heavy bleeding.

GLOSSARY

DYSMENORRHOEA Painful periods. Primary dysmenorrhoea (no underlying disease process) is common and can be treated/supported. Secondary dysmenorrhoea is due to disease process like endometriosis or adenomyosis.

DYSPAREUNIA Pain during sex.

ECTOPIC PREGNANCY A pregnancy developing outside of the uterus, typically the fallopian tubes. This is a medical emergency.

ENDOCRINE SYSTEM Hormonal system within the body: our organs produce hormones (ovaries, pituitary, thyroid, etc) such as oestrogen, adrenaline, cortisol, etc.

ENDOMETRIAL HYPERPLASIA Thickening of the uterus lining (endometrium) due to unopposed oestrogen or dysfunction in the menstrual cycle. Can increase the risk of endometrial cancer.

ENDOMETRIOMA A cyst filled with blood (often called a chocolate cyst) seen in endometriosis, situated on the ovary.

ENDOMETRIOSIS Incurable condition when endometrial-like tissue grows outside of the uterus, causing pain, infertility and scarring. Has the potential to cause organ damage and is a disease process of endocrine and immune dysfunction.

ENDOMETRIUM The inner lining of the uterus that thickens during the menstrual cycle, with the outer layer shedding to form the period each cycle.

EXCISION SURGERY A surgical procedure used to treat endometriosis where endometriotic lesions are 'cut out' rather than burned.

FIBROIDS Benign uterine growths (tumours) growing in different layers of the uterus. Can cause heavy bleeding, pain and infertility.

FOLLICLE A fluid-filled sac in the ovary containing a developing egg.

FSH (Follicle Stimulating Hormone) A hormone produced by the pituitary to stimulate the ovaries as part of the menstrual cycle.

GnRH ANALOGUES Medications that supress ovarian hormones to induce a temporary menopause state.

GSM (Genitourinary Syndrome of Menopause) Umbrella term for the vaginal, vulval and urinary symptoms seen in menopause due to low oestrogen levels.

HIRSUTISM The term used to describe excessive hair growth in a male-pattern distribution due to higher androgens (male hormones).

GLOSSARY

HMB (Heavy Menstrual Bleeding) Bleeding in periods that is in excess of a healthy/expected amount.

HORMONES Chemical messengers that control processes within the body such as menstrual cycles, metabolism, etc. Oestrogen and progesterone are female-linked hormones used to regulate the menstrual cycle and fertility.

HRT (Hormone Replacement Therapy) Artificial hormones delivered in medications (oral tablets, patches, vaginal rings) to replace hormones lost during menopause such as oestrogen and progesterone. Given to relieve menopausal symptoms and for longer-term health protection.

HYPOMENORRHOEA Abnormally light periods, blood loss <35mls during the cycle or a period lasting two days or less.

IUD (Intrauterine device, commonly called the coil hypomenorrhoea) A copper IUD is non-hormonal and the IUS is a hormone-based coil. Used for contraceptive purposes.

IUI (Intrauterine Insemination) A method of ART fertility support where the sperm is inserted into the uterus with medical assistance to help achieve a pregnancy.

IUS (Intrauterine system, commonly called the hormonal coil) Hormone-based IUD, levonorgestrel-releasing device for contraceptive purposes or to reduce bleeding, pain and protect the endometrium.

IVF (In Vitro Fertilization) The term used for fertility medicine (ART) for intervention to support a pregnancy. The egg is harvested and fertilized by sperm 'in vitro' (in a controlled setting) and the fertilized embryo is inserted into the uterus.

LAPAROSCOPY Keyhole surgery to diagnose or treat conditions within the abdomen or pelvis.

LAPAROTOMY Surgical procedure where the abdomen is opened with a longer incision (different and higher risk to laparoscopy). Less commonly used in period-related management pathways.

LH (Luteinizing Hormone) The hormone involved in menstrual cycles to trigger ovulation.

LICHEN SCLEROSIS An autoimminue skin condition affecting the vulva, causing itching, soreness, ulcerations and scarring. It is a premalignant condition that requires treatment with topical steroids and correct management to reduce risk of vulva cancer.

LUTEAL PHASE The part of the menstrual cycle after ovulation; progesterone levels are high in this phase.

MENOPAUSE The twelve months after the final period.

MENORRHAGIA Heavy menstrual bleeding, can be primary (no underlying disease process) or secondary (due to an underlying disease such as fibroids).

MITTELSCHMERZ A term sometimes used in medicine to describe period pain associated with ovulation.

NORETHISTERONE A synthetic progesterone hormone (progestogen) used in management of period-related conditions or as a contraceptive. Often used to temporarily delay periods.

OESTROGEN Female hormone used for ovulation, regulation of cycles and influencing libido and female characteristics (breasts, fat distribution). Also important for bone and heart health.

OLIGOMENORRHOEA Infrequent periods (cycles that are longer than 35 days).

OVULATION The release of an egg during the menstrual cycle.

PCOS (Polycystic Ovary Syndrome) A condition where there is irregular ovulation and higher androgens (testosterone), causing hirsutism features and metabolic changes (insulin resistance).

PERIMENOPAUSE The time leading up to menopause where hormones fluctuate and symptoms begin to appear.

PERITONEUM Anatomical name for the membrane (thin tissue) lining that covers the abdominal organs.

PMDD (Premenstrual Dysphoric Disorder) A severe form of PMS causing significant mood changes including severe anxiety, depression or suicidal thoughts.

PMS (Premenstrual Syndrome) The term used for physical and emotional symptoms arising from hormone fluctuations during the menstrual cycle. Often seen during the luteal phase.

POSTMENOPAUSE The time after Peritoneum menopause (i.e. 12 months have elapsed). During this time any bleeding would be considered a red flag and needs investigation.

PROGESTERONE The natural hormone that works alongside oestrogen to maintain the menstrual cycle. Responsible for the uterine lining and support in early pregnancy.

PROGESTOGEN The synthetic form of progesterone used in hormone-based medications.

TESTOSTERONE An androgen hormone, responsible for male characteristics. Those with PCOS will usually have higher levels.

UTERUS Also referred to as the womb, the central part of the reproductive organs that produces a period and hosts a pregnancy. Consists of three layers: the muscular layer which causes contractions and the inner layer, the endometrium, which thickens during the cycle and sheds to produce a period in the absence of a pregnancy.

VAGINA The internal muscular canal that can't be seen and leads from the vulva to the cervix (where the tampon sits).

VULVA The external anatomy that is visible, including the labia, clitoris, urethral opening and vaginal opening.

REFERENCES

CHAPTERS 1–3

- European Society of Human Reproduction and Embryology ESHRE (2022) | ESHRE Endometriosis Guideline Development Group (2022) 'Endometriosis Guideline of European Society of Human Reproduction and Embryology' (Accessed online, 2025)
- ESHRE (2024) Premature Ovarian Insufficiency (POI) Guideline of European Society of Human Reproduction and Embryology (Accessed online, 2025)
- Medicines & Healthcare Products Regulatory Agency (2020) 'Measuring the incidence and prevalence of menstrual disorders in the UK Clinical Practice Research Datalink', (Accessed online, 2025)
- House of Commons, Women and Equalities Committee (2024–25) 'Women's reproductive health conditions' First Report of Session 2024–25. (Accessed online, 2025)
- Department for Education (Jan 2022) 'Period Products Scheme – Ad-hoc statistics: 2021 Management Information' (Accessed online, 2025)
- NICE National Institute for Health and Care Excellence (Published 2019, Updated 2021), 'Heavy Menstrual Bleeding: Assessment and Management', full guideline (Accessed online, 2025)
- NICE Guidelines Online, National Institute for Health and Care Excellence, Nov 2024, Health Topics A to Z > Menorrhagia, https://cks.nice.org.uk/topics/menorrhagia-heavy-menstrual-bleeding/ (Accessed online, 2025)
- NICE Guidelines Online, National Institute for Health and Care Excellence, Nov 2024, Health Topics A to Z > Menorrhagia, https://www.nice.org.uk/guidance/ng88 (Accessed online, 2025)
- National Institute for Health and Care Excellence (2018) Dysmenorrhoea: Clinical Knowledge Summary 2014
- National Institute for Health and Care Excellence (2018) Heavy menstrual bleeding: assessment and management

REFERENCES

- Public Health England (online) 'Health Inequalities: Menstrual Issues' (Accessed online, 2025)
- Royal College General Practitioners (2025) 'Women's Health Toolkit – Menstrual Health', https://elearning.rcgp.org.uk/mod/book/view.php?id=12534&chapterid=819 (Accessed online, 2025)
- Marjoribanks, J et al (2016) 'Surgery Versus Medical Therapy for Heavy Menstrual Bleeding', Cochrane Library, Jan 29;2016(1):CD003855 doi: 10.1002/14651858. CD003855.pub3, https://pubmed.ncbi.nlm.nih.gov/26820670/ (Accessed online, 2025)
- Hill, S. *How The Pill Changes Everything* 2019, Penguin Random House
- Bashiri A, Halper KI, Orvieto R. Recurrent Implantation Failure-update overview on etiology, diagnosis, treatment and future directions. *Reprod Biol Endocrinol*. 2018 Dec 5;16(1):121. doi: 10.1186/s12958-018-0414-2. PMID: 30518389; PMCID: PMC 6282265
- Gildersleeve K, Haselton MG, Fales MR. Do women's mate preferences change across the ovulatory cycle? A meta-analytic review. *Psychol Bull*. 2014 Sep;140(5):1205-59. doi: 10.1037/a0035438. Epub 2014 Feb 24. PMID: 24564172.
- Peters M, Simmons LW, Rhodes G. Preferences across the menstrual cycle for masculinity and symmetry in photographs of male faces and bodies. *Plos one*. 2009 ;4(1):e4138. DOI: 10.1371/journal.pone.0004138. PMID: 19127295; PMCID: PMC2607552.

CHAPTERS 4–8

- Morotti, M et al (Feb 2017) 'Mechanisms of pain in endometriosis', *European Journal of Obstetrics & Gynaecology and Reproductive Biology*, Volume 209, pages 8-13. (Accessed online, 2025)
- Cano-Herrera et al. (2024) 'Endometriosis: A Comprehensive Analysis of the Pathophysiology, Treatment, and Nutritional Aspects, and Its Repercussions on the Quality of Life of Patients', *Biomedicines*, 2024 Jul 4;12(7): 1476. (Accessed online, PubMed Central 2025)

REFERENCES

- Horne, Andrew et al. (2022) 'Pathophysiology, diagnosis, and management of endometriosis', *BMJ* 2022;379:e070750 doi: https://doi.org/10.1136/bmj-2022-070750 (Accessed online, 2025)
- Zhang, H et al. (2023) 'Immune and endocrine regulation in endometriosis: What we know', *Journal of Endometriosis and Uterine Disorders*, Vol 4, 100049 https://doi.org/10.1016/j.jeud.2023.100049 (Accessed via Science Direct Online, 2025)
- Liang, Y et al. (2016) 'Potential role of estrogen in maintaining the imbalanced sympathetic and sensory innervation in endometriosis', *Molecular and Cellular Endocrinology*, Vol 424, March 2026, Pages 42-49 DOI: https://doi.org/10.1016/j.mce.2016.01.012 (Accessed online via Science Direct, 2025)
- World Health Organisation online resources 'Endometriosis' (March 2023) https://www.who.int/news-room/fact-sheets/detail/endometriosis (Accessed online, 2025)
- Yang S et al. (2011) 'Progesterone: the ultimate endometrial tumor suppressor', *Trends In Endocrinology & Metabolism*, Vol 22, Issue 4 Pages 145-152 DOI https://doi.org/10.1016/j.tem.2011.01.005 (Accessed Online via Science Direct, 2025)
- Royal College of Obstetricians and Gynaecologists (2006) 'The Investigation and Management of Endometriosis', Green-top Guideline No. 24 Oct 2006
- O Burney R. et al. (2012) 'Pathogenesis and Pathophysiology of Endometriosis', *Fertil Steril* Jul 20;98(3):10.1016 doi:10.1016/j.fertnstert.2012.06.029 (Accessed online via Pubmed, 2025)
- Zito, G et al. (2014) 'Medical Treatments for Endometriosis-Associated Pelvic Pain', *Biomedical Research International*. Aug 7;2014:191967 doi: 10.1155/2014/191967 (Access online via Pubmed, 2025)
- Monnin, N et al. (2023) 'Endometriosis: Update of Pathophysiology, (Epi) Genetic and Environmental Involvement' *Biomedicines*. March 22;11(3): 978 doi: 10.3390/biomedicines11030978 (Accessed online via Pubmed, 2025)
- Capezzuoli, T et al. (2022) 'Hormonal Drugs For the Treatment of Endometriosis' *Current Opinion in Pharmacology*, Vol 67, 102311 DOI: https://doi.org/10.1016/j.coph.2022.102311 (Accessed online via Science Direct, 2025)
- Vaannuccini, S et al. (2021) 'Hormonal Treatments For Endometriosis: The endocrine background', *Rev Endocr Metabl Disord*. 2021 Aug 17;23(3):333-355 doi: 10.1007/s11154-021-09666-w (Accessed online via Pubmed, 2025)

REFERENCES

- Pasalic E, et al. (2023) 'Endometriosis: Classification, pathophysiology, and treatment options', *Pathology – Research and Practice* 251 (2023) 154847 (Accessed online via Science Direct, 2025)
- Taniguchi, F et al. (2015) 'Effects of low dose oral contraceptive pill containing drospirenone/ethinylestradiol in patients with endometrioma' *European Journal of Obstetrics & Gynaecology and Reproductive Biology*, Vol 191, 116-120 https://doi.org/10.1016/j.ejogrb.2015.06.006 (Accessed online via Science Direct, 2025)
- Women Living Better (2024) 'Progesterone and Progestins' https://womenlivingbetter.org/progesterone-and-progestins/
- Cable, J et al. (2023) 'Physiology, Progesterone' StatPearls (internet) (Accessed online via Pubmed, 2025)

CHAPTERS 9–12

- NICE Guidelines Online, National Institute for Health and Care Excellence, April 2023, Health Topics A to Z > Fibroids, https://cks.nice.org.uk/topics/fibroids/ (Accessed online, 2025)
- NICE Guidelines Online, National Institute for Health and Care Excellence, March 2025, Health Topics A to Z > Polycystic Ovary Syndrome, https://cks.nice.org.uk/topics/polycystic-ovary-syndrome/ (Accessed online, 2025)
- NICE Guidelines Online, National Institute for Health and Care Excellence, July 2025, Health Topics A to Z >Premature Ovarian Insufficiency https://cks.nice.org.uk/topics/menopause/diagnosis/diagnosis-of-premature-ovarian-insufficiency/ (Accessed online, 2025)
- NICE Guidelines Online, National Institute for Health and Care Excellence, July 2025, Health Topics A to Z >Menopause https://cks.nice.org.uk/topics/menopause/ (Accessed online, 2025)
- Cannon, E. *The Little* Book of HRT, 2025, Green Tree Publishers

ACKNOWLEDGEMENTS

Thank you to my two children, who have made me the woman I am today and kept me focused on always striving to be the best version of myself, for choosing me to be your mama and being there with love and open arms unconditionally. You are the essence of joy and have been my guiding light even when you didn't realize it. I am so grateful for your patience with me while I try to work towards a solid future for us. I have always tried to work around you and put your needs first but know there were days when I was tired and I thank you for your patience as well as your interest in what it is I do. Know that everything I do, I do for our family, our future and also for your generation. I hope one day you appreciate my efforts in trying to share my personal and professional experiences so that those in your world don't have to endure as many of the challenges my generation did.

Thank you to dad for being there to help pick up the flack when I have needed to bunker down in my cave and for humouring my relentless aspirations, dreams and passions for wanting to take what I've gone through and make it into something better for someone else. I truly appreciate the hours you have given to allow me to work, travel and pursue my dreams.

A huge thank you to Tor and Ed – for both seeing in me my potential and giving me a huge helping hand to take the next steps. You have always been there full of smiles, encouragement and honesty and I am forever grateful for your part in my journey and being incredible friends.

Thank you to Sammy, Pam and my fellow team behind the charity. For being patient as I share my time writing and pursuing my intentions with striving for change in women's health and humouring my endless voice notes and ramblings. Sammy, you have been such a big part of this chapter of my life and I thank you for bringing SOG to life with me.

Thank you to all my friends and in particular Looly and Laura for having my back and keeping me going in life and work the past few years. You make me laugh, keep me grounded, help me enjoy life and I am so grateful to you. To Amy,

ACKNOWLEDGEMENTS

up there in the heavens looking down – I hope you know how much I appreciate your time in my life and you were such an amazing friend and helped me believe in myself and what I wanted to achieve. I am forever grateful for your short time on this Earth and that I was lucky to have had you as a friend.

Thank you to Ele – my E^2 – for being the tortoise to my hare and keeping me from sprinting too fast, bringing the smile back to my life and being such a champion to my work, energy and ideas. You have shown me the deepest of joys I never believed possible and I am forever grateful to have you by my side.

Such sincere thanks to my incredible editors Katie, Jo and all the team at Octopus for everything you have done with the book, the cover and helping me bring this book to life. For patiently reading my enthusiastic ramblings, helping me channel these thoughts and ideas and delivering this book to fruition. You have been the best team to work with for my debut book and have made it such a joyous experience. Thank you to all the team involved in the cover for giving a face to something so personal.

Thank you to my amazing agent Jo – I could not have asked for a better agent. Thank you for seeing me, seeing my ideas and believing in what I want to share in my work. Your guidance, patient cheerleading and sharing the joy along the way with me has made this experience wonderful. I am so grateful for your trust, support and enthusiasm.

And finally, a thank you to every woman and patient who has ever allowed me to be their doctor, confidante, friend, advisor, counsellor or friendly ear. I have listened to every single one of you, seen your journey and taken notes along the way. Right from being a medical student. Even if I couldn't help you at the time, I was listening and trying to find a way to help in some way, at some point. I hope this book helps each of you in the way I want it to.

INDEX

adenomyomectomy 207
adenomyosis 10–11, 43, 47, 49, 53, 58, 86, 201–10
    diagnosis 204–5
    and endometriosis 201–2, 203
    and hysterectomy 232
    and PD (primary dysmenorrhoea) 64, 66
ADHD 256–7
adrogens
    and PCOS 211, 213, 214
AI misinformation 4, 7
amenorrhoea (absence of periods) 49, 59
angiogenesis 89
anorexia 49
antidepressants 58, 111–12, 151
anxiety 55
aromatase inhibitors 157, 161–2, 218
ART (assisted reproductive technology) 176–8, 181–3, 208–9, 216–18, 261
autoimmune diseases 93–5, 113–14, 174, 222

biopsies
    diagnosing endometriosis 134
birth trauma 4
bladder changes
    and endometriosis 86, 170
bloating
    and endometriosis 108–9
bowel
    and endometriosis 86, 106–7, 170
    IBS (irritable bowel syndrome) 105–6
    stoma 107

cancer
    endometrial 220, 230, 232
    gynaeological cancers 11, 21–2
    and the immune system 89
    ovarian 86, 87
    uterine 47, 49, 214
    vulva 237, 238
cardiovascular health 239
cervix 20, 21, 22, 26
chemical pregnancies 30
childhood 22
clomifene 217–18
community support 256
contraception 155, 215
contraceptive pill 10, 32, 37, 75
    and endometriosis 107, 115, 126, 130, 139, 155
    and fibroids 197
    and menopause 229
    and menstrual disorders 66, 67, 68–9
    and PCOS 219
Cox enzymes 63
Cox inhibitors 65–6

depression 55, 104, 109
diabetes 215, 216, 222
diet and well-being 254–5
dietary supplements 242
disability and endometriosis 119
disenfranchised grief 139
DUB (dysfunctional uterine bleeding) 47, 48
dysmenorrhoea (painful periods) 40, 43–4, 44, 49–55, 58–9, 60
    and adenomyosis 202
    and endometriosis 51, 52–3, 54, 64, 66, 67, 78, 103, 121, 130
    and fibroids 186
    misperception as 'normal' 2, 4–5, 6, 7, 8
    primary 50–3, 54, 61, 62–7, 70
    secondary 53–5, 61

INDEX

ectopic pregnancies 54
education
   girls and periods 37–8
eggs 21
   donation 225
   fertilization 30
   freezing 176
   ovulation 27–9
embryos 30
   freezing 179–80
emergency toolkit for flares 256
employers 118
endocrine disorders 49, 83–4
endocrine system 89–92
endometrial ablation 198, 207
endometrial cancer 220, 230, 232
endometrial plaques 82, 83, 85–6, 87–8
   and the bowel 106–7
   and hormonal treatments 164
   and infertility 173
   and oestrogen 89, 90
   and pain 91, 103–4
   and stages of endometriosis 98–9
endometriosis 1, 6, 10, 11, 17, 23, 43, 47, 49, 58, 73–185
   and adenomyosis 201–2, 203
   causes of 80–1
   counselling for 262–3
   diagnosis 121–44
      'suspected endometriosis' 136–9
      suspected to confirmed 139–41
   and dysmenorrhoea 51, 52–3, 54, 64, 66, 67, 78
   fertility and pregnancy 171–84
   history of 78–9
   and hysterectomy 232
   and the immune system 51, 52–3, 54, 64, 66, 67, 78, 79
   living with 101–20, 260–1
   management and treatment 121, 135, 136, 145–70
      GnRH analogues 157, 159–63, 169
      hormonal treatments 152–65, 169
      medication v. surgery 149–50
      obstacles to 147–9
      relugolix 162–3
      surgery 166–9
   medical pathways explained 122–3
   NICE guidelines for 118
   physiology of 88–96
   and quality of life 118–19
   reasons for misunderstanding of 79–80
   rebound endometriosis 163–4
   science of 84–8
   secondary health conditions 81
   secondary (hospital) care 123, 137
   social stigma of 75
   stages of 96–9
   symptoms and signs of 101–3
endometrium 26–7, 29, 30, 39
   and adenomyosis 202
   and endometriosis 81, 82, 84–5
   and fibroids 189
Esmya 197

fallopian tubes 20, 21, 29
   and endometriosis 82, 86
female anatomy 18–22
fertility 10, 16
   and adenomyosis 204, 208–9
   the fertile years 23
   fibroids 192
   issues with 3
   and PCOS 212–14, 216–18
   and POI 220–1, 225
   symptoms 191–2
   treatments 176–83
   see also infertility
fibroids 10–11, 43, 46, 47, 48, 49, 53, 60, 61, 129, 154, 185–200
   and adenomyosis 203, 204–5
   diagnosis 194–5
   intramural 190
   management options 195–9

subserosal 191, 192
submucosal 190, 191, 192
symptoms 184, 191–3
FSH (follicle-stimulating hormone) 25, 29

genetics
and endometriosis 80
GnRH (gonadotropin-releasing hormone)
analogues/agonists 25, 157,
159–63, 169, 197, 232
GP appointments 9
diagnosing endometriosis 123, 126–9,
136–9, 140, 142
diagnosing fibroids 194–5
grief process 223, 248–9
disenfranchised grief 139
GSM (genitourinary syndrome) 236

hCG (pregnancy hormone) 30, 174
health
periods as markers of 8–9
hirsutism 213, 216, 219
HMB (heavy menstrual bleeding)
causes of 46–7
hormone treatments
for adenomyosis 206–7
for endometriosis 114–15, 130
for menstrual disorders 69
hormones 10, 261
and endometriosis 79, 83–4
hormone sensitivity 32–3
and the immune system 95–6
and the menstrual cycle 17, 18, 22, 24–6
and physical attraction 31
HRT (hormone replacement therapy) 155,
168, 188
and hysterectomy 232
and menopause 233, 239, 240–2, 244
and PCOS 220
hypermobility 117–18, 257
hysterectomy 6, 11, 77, 231–2
and adenomyosis 205, 207, 210

and endometriosis 107, 167–9
and fibroids 199
and menopause 241

iatrogenic POI 221, 222
IBS (irritable bowel syndrome) 105–6
ICE method of communication 127, 130,
253–4
identity 5, 12
immune system 113–14
and endometriosis 51, 52–3, 54, 64, 66,
67, 78, 79, 83–4, 88–9, 92–6, 173
infertility 70
and adenomyosis 201
and endometriosis 78, 81, 101–2, 110,
168, 172–4
secondary 4, 30, 94, 172–3
see also fertility
insomnia 236
insulin resistance 215, 225
IUDs/IUSs 47, 54, 69, 105
IUI (intrauterine insemination) 208
IVF 6, 77, 84, 172, 178–83, 193, 208–9,
222, 261

laparoscopy
endometriosis 70, 121, 123, 133–5, 139,
166–7, 169
fibroids 195
letrozole 218
LH (luteinizing hormone) 25, 29
life-changing disease, living with 245–6
relationship impact 251–2
LS (lichen sclerosis) 237–8
LUNA (laparoscopic uterosacral nerve
ablation) 169
lupus 93, 94–5

medications
and endometriosis 111–12
and menstrual disorders 47, 49
menarche 23

INDEX

menopause 5, 10, 16, 32, 227–44, 262
  age of 229–30
  bleeding after menopause 41
  bone health 238–9
  chemical 112, 159–60, 232–3
  defining 24
  early 3, 11, 230
  and fibroids 199
  impact of 233–4
  and mood disorders 58
  and PCOS 219–20
  and POI 222, 225
  post-menopausal bleeding 230
  premature 228, 230–1, 238–9
  surgical 112, 168, 231–2
  symptoms 234–7
  types of 229–33
menorrhagia (heavy periods) 46, 48, 49, 58–9, 60
  and adenomyosis 202
  and fibroids 186, 189, 191
  primary 61, 67–71
  secondary 61
menstrual cycle/menstruation 15–17, 35–60
  absence of 214–15
  changes over time 41
  cultural attitudes to 1–2
  dysfunctional 9
  healthy periods 8–9, 39–42
  myths around 9
  period health 42
  in puberty 5, 35
  reasons for 17, 29–31
  retrograde menstruation 80–1
  taboos around 1
  timing of the menstrual cycle 29
  understanding your periods 15–17
menstrual disorders 9, 44–60
  amenorrhoea (absence of periods) 49, 59
  markers of unhealthy periods 42–4
  metrorrhagia (irregular bleeding) 49, 52, 214–15
  mood-related problems 55–8

oligomenorrhoea (infrequent bleeding) 49
  see also dysmenorrhoea (painful periods); menorrhagia (heavy periods)
menstrual flow 27, 39–40
  heavy periods 32–4, 38, 39, 43–4
  normalizing 2, 4–5, 6, 7, 8, 35–6
  primary causes of 9
  vaginal discharge 40
menstrual products 9
  advertising 1
Mental and Strong (charity) 246
mental well-being 249–50
metformin 218
metrorrhagia (irregular bleeding) 49, 52, 214–15
micro-traumas 249, 250–1
miscarriages 4, 6, 30, 77, 82, 83, 84, 94, 110, 174–5, 204
mood 10, 40–1
  disorders 41
  and endometriosis 109, 115–16
  and hormone sensitivity 32–3
  and menstrual disorders 44, 55–8
myomectomy 197
myometrium 26

neurodiversity 256–7
  and endometriosis 116, 117–18
neurogenesis 89
NICE guidelines
  diagnosing endometriosis 123, 128, 132
  for endometriosis 118
nosebleeds 87
NSAIDs (non-steroidal anti-inflammatories) 65, 69, 206

oestrogen 16, 40–1
  and adenomyosis 204
  and endometriosis 82, 84, 85, 87, 89–92, 96, 115–16, 117
  treatment 152, 153, 154, 155, 156–7, 158
  impact of 31–3
  and menopause 236–7, 238–9, 243–4

and the menstrual cycle 22, 25
and mood 55
and pain 89–92, 110
and POI 222
oligomenorrhoea (infrequent bleeding) 49
oocytes 27, 38
osteoporosis 238–9, 242
ovarian cancer 86, 87
ovaries 20, 21, 86
POI (primary ovarian insufficiency) 211, 220–4, 225
ovulation 25–6, 39, 40, 174

pain
 and endometriosis 88, 89–92, 96–8, 103–5, 109, 260
 and the bowel 106
 and oestrogen 90–1, 96, 97
 pain relief 92
pain relief
 and endometriosis 111–12, 129–30, 136, 145, 148–9, 150–2
painful periods *see* dysmenorrhoea (painful periods)
patient advocates 10
PCOS (polycystic ovary syndrome) 10–11, 49, 59, 211–20, 224–5
 diagnosis 211–13
PD (primary dysmenorrhoea) 50–3, 54, 61, 62–7, 70
pelvic inflammatory disease 54
perimenopause 22–4, 229, 233
periods *see* dysmenorrhoea (painful periods); menstrual cycle/menstruation; menstrual flow
peritoneum 88
PIF (Patient Information Forum) 254
PM (primary menorrhagia) 61, 67–71
PMDD (premenstrual dysphoric disorder) 56–7, 59, 256, 257
 and endometriosis 116, 118
PMS (premenstrual syndrome) 56, 57, 59
 and endometriosis 116, 118

POI (primary ovarian insufficiency) 211, 220–4, 225
post-menopause 24
postnatal depression 175, 256
postnatal mood disorders 57
pregnancy
 and adenomyosis 202, 204–5, 209
 caesarean sections 209
 ectopic pregnancies 54
 and endometriosis treatment 159
 fertilization and implantation 27
 and fibroids 192
 and the menstrual cycle 25, 26
 and POI 224
 vaginal bleeding 87
presacral neurectomy 169
primary dysmenorrhoea (PD) 50–3, 54, 61, 62–7, 70
progesterone 16, 40–1
 and endometriosis 82, 85, 87, 115–16, 117
  treatment 153, 154, 155, 156–7, 158–9
 and fertility treatment 197
 impact of 31–3
 and the menstrual cycle 22, 25–6
 and mood 55, 56
prostaglandins 62–3, 65, 67
PTSD (post-traumatic stress disorder) 250
puberty 5, 22–3, 38, 228, 263–4

quality of life
 and endometriosis 118–19

relugolix 162–3

scans 132–3, 136, 188
 and adenomyosis 204
self-help 254–8
sex
 orgasm 104, 111
 pain during 104–5, 110–11
 and surgical menopause 112

sex education in schools 7
'shoulding' 265–6
social media misinformation 4
sperm
   and ovulation 29
   spoon theory 246–8, 249
surgery
   adenomyosis 207
   fibroid removal 197–8
   hysterectomy 167–9
   prior to IVF 179
   see also hysterectomy; laparoscopy
symptom diaries 70

tranexamic acid 69, 206

UAE (uterine artery embolization) 198
uterine cancer 47, 49, 214
uterus 19, 20, 21
   adenomyosis 201–10
   and endometriosis 86, 128–9

vagina 20, 21, 26
   menopause and vaginal health 241, 243
vulva 19, 21, 22
vulva cancer 237, 238

weight gain
   and endometriosis 108–9, 117
weight loss 217, 218
womanhood, stages of 22–4

ABOUT THE AUTHOR

DR LIZ MURRAY
BCA(H), MBBS, Dip MedSci

Dr Liz Murray is a British medical doctor, author and women's health advocate specializing in menstrual health, chronic gynaecological conditions and patient-led healthcare reform.

A former NHS doctor, she bridges clinical expertise with lived experience to address the widespread normalization of menstrual pain and delayed diagnosis in women's healthcare. Her work focuses on conditions including endometriosis, adenomyosis, PCOS, premature ovarian insufficiency and PMDD.

After navigating her own health challenges including autoimmune disease, endometriosis, secondary infertility and a hysterectomy in her early thirties, Liz began utilizing her unique insight as both patient and doctor to strive for patient-centric care reform.

Liz is the founder of the charity Mortal And Strong, which supports individuals navigating complex diagnoses and recovery from serious illness, and leads public education initiatives on health equity and patient empowerment.

For her work as an activist addressing health inequalities, Liz was the recipient of the British Citizen Award (People's Honours) for her services to health.

Through writing, speaking and media commentary, Liz works to improve understanding of menstrual health as a vital component of whole-body wellbeing.

FURTHER RESOURCES

Further Support

Here are some other useful resources and materials I would recommend to anyone wanting to know about some of these topics.

Patient Information Forum

The Patient Information Forum (PIF) is the UK's only regulatory body for providing assurance of reliable health information, particularly online. Regulation of online health advice is not yet legally mandatory in the UK, but most reputable charities, organisations and independent health advocates or public-facing doctors are voluntarily regulated. The PIF TICK is an indicator that the information you are seeing is reliable, produced to a safe standard for providing evidence-based information. Their website has a list of all the organisations and individuals who are PIF-Ticked (myself included) which would always be somewhere I would advise going to for reassurance that what you are reading is reliable.

Websites

NHS (NHS.uk)

The online NHS website provides reliable, up to date information about most health conditions, including expected treatments, investigations and processes.

NICE (NICE.org.uk)

The National Institute for Health and Care Excellence (NICE) provides guidelines for clinicians based on the latest evidence-based research and information. Intended for doctors, but patients can always use their website to find out the recommended pathways and processes to help in any discussions about their care.

ENDO1000 (Endo1000.com)

A research project striving for improving the diagnosis pathway for endometriosis, but their website provides a lot of reliable information. There are also potential calls for volunteers to assist in research.

RCOG (rcog.org.uk)
The Royal College of Obstetricians & Gynaecologists (RCOG) is the medical institution that overseas training and assessments of consultants specialising in O&G. Their website also provides information for patients which is reliable, evidence based and up to date.

Fertility Network UK (fertilitynetworkuk.org)
A charity providing support and information for people facing fertility challenges.

HFEA (hfea.gov.uk)
Human Fertilisation & Embryology Authority (HFEA UK) is the UK's fertility regulator. Couples seeking impartial and reliable information about treatments or fertility clinics, this is a highly recommended starting place.

World Endometriosis Society (worldendosociety.org)
An international organisation providing guidance, research and advanced standards in endometriosis care. Their work focuses on improving the standard of care and research for endometriosis, and their website contains reliable, up to date information on endometriosis.

Books

The Vagina Bible **by Dr Jen Gunter**
A brilliant book providing a vast amount of information to help women understand their vulva from their vagina and the many ways in which our lives can impact our reproductive health. A brilliant read.

The Little Book of HRT **by DR Ellie Cannon**
A useful book providing detailed information about all different areas of hormone treatments and menopause.

Contraception **by Alice Pelton, Dr Frances Yarlett & Dr Melanie Davis-Hall**
A reliable guide covering all aspects of all the various contraceptives, separating fact from fiction.

Taking a book from manuscript to market is a team effort. This book was carefully created by

Publisher: Jo Morrell
Commissioning Editor: Katie Forsythe
Project Editor: Rimsha Falak
Copy Editor: Emma Bastow
Designer: Rachael Shone
Editorial Assistant: Sarah Ramnath-Budhram
Production Controller: Sarah Parry
Sales: Lucy Helliwell & Rachel Lowth
Marketing & Publicity: Erin Brown & Chloë Johnson-Hill

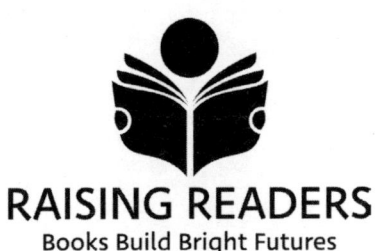

RAISING READERS
Books Build Bright Futures

Dear Reader,

We'd love your attention for one more page to tell you about the crisis in children's reading, and what we can all do.

Studies have shown that reading for fun is the **single biggest predictor of a child's future life chances** – more than family circumstance, parents' educational background or income. It improves academic results, mental health, wealth, communication skills, ambition and happiness.[1]

The number of children reading for fun is in rapid decline. Young people have a lot of competition for their time. In 2024, 1 in 10 children and young people in the UK aged 5 to 18 did not own a single book at home.[2]

Hachette works extensively with schools, libraries and literacy charities, but here are some ways we can all raise more readers:

- Reading to children for just 10 minutes a day makes a difference
- Don't give up if children aren't regular readers – there will be books for them!
- Visit bookshops and libraries to get recommendations
- Encourage them to listen to audiobooks
- Support school libraries
- Give books as gifts

There's a lot more information about how to encourage children to read on our website: **www.RaisingReaders.co.uk**

Thank you for reading.

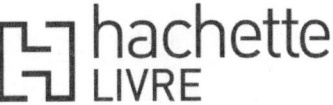

---

[1] OECD, '21st-Century Readers: Developing Literacy Skills in a Digital World', 2021, https://www.oecd.org/en/publications/21st-century-readers_a83d84cb-en.html

[2] National Literacy Trust, 'Book Ownership in 2024', November 2024, https://literacytrust.org.uk/research-services/research-reports/book-ownership-in-2024